HEALTH & WE

Pilates

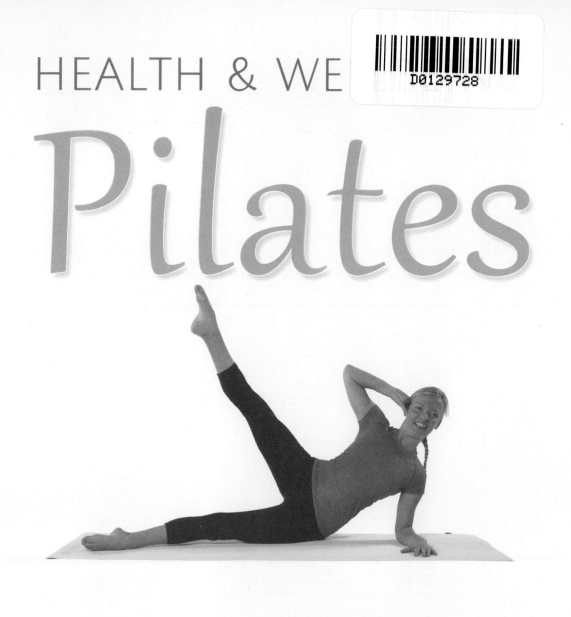

This is a **FLAME TREE** book
First published 2013

Publisher and Creative Director: Nick Wells
Senior Project Editor: Catherine Taylor
Copy Editor: Anna Groves
Editorial and Picture Research: Esme Chapman and Emma Chafer
Art Director and Layout Design: Mike Spender
Photographer: Alexandra Hunt
Photography Director: Charmaine Yabsley
Proofreader: Dawn Laker
Indexer: Helen Snaith

Acknowledgements

With many thanks to several people who worked long and hard to produce such a beautiful book. We would like to express our thanks to Indianna Franke, a Pilates instructor and physiotherapist who took the time to advise on the exercises in the book as well as to pose so wonderfully for our photographs. Indianna, along with her husband Radd Peters, own The Living Well Studio. Visit www.thelivingwellstudio.com.au

We would also like to thank Lululemon Clothing for the loan of their Pilates gear. Visit www.lululemon.com.au

With many thanks to Alexandra Hunt for her fantastic photographs.

The author would also like to express her many thanks to the editor, Catherine Taylor, for her help and guidance with this project.

Publisher's Note:

This edition first published 2013 by
FLAME TREE PUBLISHING
Crabtree Hall, Crabtree Lane
Fulham, London SW6 6TY
United Kingdom

www.flametreepublishing.com

ISBN 978-0-85775-997-9

A CIP record for this book is available from the British Library upon request.

HEALTH & WELLBEING

Pilates

Charmaine Yabsley

Foreword by Katy Louise Evans,
Editor of Bodyfit magazine

**FLAME TREE
PUBLISHING**

Contents

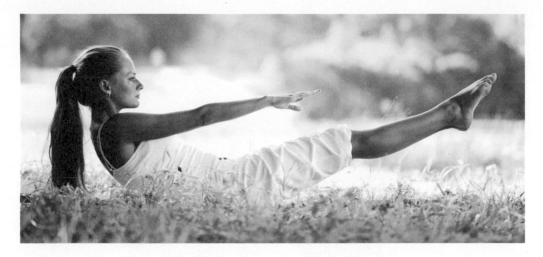

Pilates has so much to offer both the body and mind that making this discipline a part of your daily routine is a great stepping stone towards a healthy lifestyle. With benefits ranging from toned muscles and improved posture through to effective stress relief, it's time to embrace the Pilates trend! Begin by learning about the history of Pilates and the ways in which it has developed since its inception. Before you start exploring the postures, it is also important to understand the six main principles of Pilates and how they underpin the practice. Discover how Classical Pilates has evolved into Modern Pilates, taking advantage of the best of both worlds.

Getting Ready

Pilates is a great form of exercise for everyone,
regardless of age, shape, size or ability level.
This section explains the variety of Pilates
classes on offer, ranging from Classical classes
to those using more complex equipment such
as the Reformer. Additionally, for those keen to
self-practise, there is all you need to know to
begin practising your routine at home, ranging
from what equipment you need to the best time
to exercise. Whether you're looking to build
bone strength, reduce back pain or just want to
introduce some mind-body connection to your
daily life, there's a Pilates option to suit you.

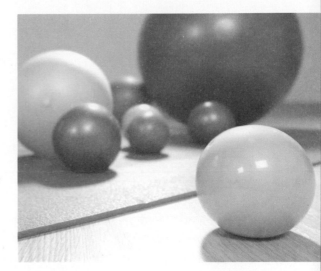

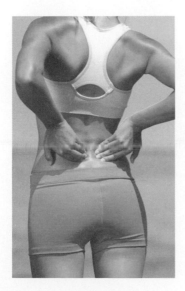

The Pilates Body

Pilates has an amazing ability to engage and improve many
areas of the human body, from top to toe. This section looks
at which areas are most involved in the Pilates movements,
and explains how you can activate your core for increased
overall strength and the benefit of other muscle groups.
Particular attention is given to the spine, which plays an
important role in stabilization and balance during any Pilates
workout. You will also learn about how to remain aware of
your lungs and diaphragm so that you can better control
your breathing 'the Pilates way', ensuring that your core
remains engaged and you get the most out of every posture.

The Exercises

With postures designed to work all the main muscle groups, the wide variety of Pilates exercises offers something for everybody. Beginning with subsections guiding you through specific types of poses – from establishing stability, through standing exercises

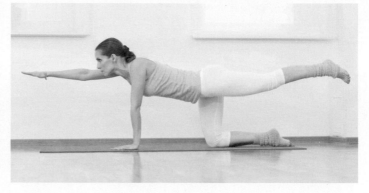

to mat postures – this chapter will see you become gradually more confident and capable in your Pilates practice until you are ready to integrate more difficult exercises into your routine and challenge your body further. Aside from a wealth of postures which range from 'Floating Arms' to 'The Hundred', you will also learn how to stretch properly and warm down effectively so that you can get the most out of every workout.

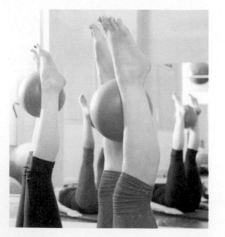

Exercises With Props

The use of props in Pilates has become increasingly popular, allowing you to challenge yourself further and help you benefit more from certain postures. The large Pilates equipment such as the Reformer, the Cadillac and the Chair are explained, before going on to the variety of different Pilates props, outlining how they work and which unique benefits they can offer. Step-by-step exercises are provided for the small ball, magic circle, Pilates ball and foam roller.

When practising Pilates, you will benefit most by considering both your ability level and what you wish to achieve, and tailoring your workout accordingly. This section covers a variety of carefully selected Pilates routines which aim to target health and fitness issues that people commonly wish to address. With workouts designed for everything from daily maintenance to toning up your bum and thighs, this section allows you to make your routine work for you. The troubleshooting subsection is a great way to ensure you know which exercises to avoid if you have certain health problems or are practising when pregnant.

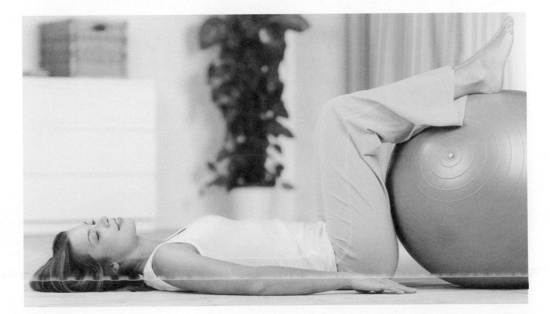

Foreword

Almost a decade ago, I attended my first Pilates class, with a fantastic Dutch teacher who taught in such a way that I'd leave her sessions feeling taller, more supple and as if my entire body had undergone a workout – though not of the ache-inducing, treadmill-pounding variety!

Sadly, my practice tailed off when the aforementioned teacher moved back to Holland, but I then sought out classes in London and attended as regularly as I could, including, more recently, warm or hot Pilates classes, where the room is heated to enable your body to relax more effectively into the postures, giving you greater benefits – and faster too!

But it's not always easy to get to a class, especially if you live out in the sticks. That's where this great new book will come in handy – and it's suitable for beginners and improvers alike. It has revived my love of Pilates and reminded me of why I need to be doing it more often.

Having trained as a ballet dancer from the age of four, I had it drummed into me to stand tall, hold my stomach in and shoulders back. I was always aware of the importance of correct alignment, not only to create graceful lines but also to maintain a healthy spine, which is the foundation of good posture. Pilates originally attracted plenty of classically trained dancers, as the classes enabled them to maintain suppleness and strength, and helped them through the rehabilitation process when they did get injured, which is a common problem for ballerinas. But you needn't be a dancer to benefit from Pilates.

Modern life often takes its toll, leading to poor posture; sitting at a computer for hours on end, as I currently do, or slumping in front of the TV, leads to tight hamstrings and hip flexors, and hunched shoulders, all of which only get worse as we age unless we take action to remedy the

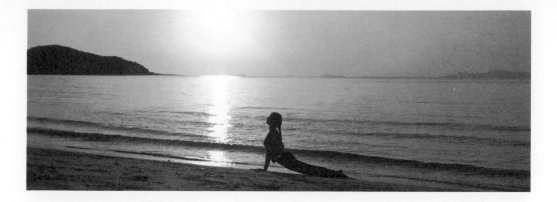

damage. Even trying to over-correct, by stiffening your back and sticking your chest out, doesn't help, as it's just as unnatural!

It's crucial we all take charge of our own bodies and wellbeing to ward off illness; Pilates, for me, is one of the best methods I know of for correcting poor posture and building a healthy fitness foundation. It can restore your vitality, strength and *joie de vivre*, not to mention increase your bone density, create stronger core muscles – meaning any back pain will be significantly reduced – tone your thighs and sculpt a pert bottom. And, if all those benefits weren't enough, Pilates can also bring you more peace of mind, thanks to the breathing techniques that help anchor your attention within your body, instead of letting the 'monkey mind' run wild, all of which is great for lowering stress levels.

In this brilliant book, Charmaine Yabsley explains the variety of classes and types of Pilates on offer, as well as how to start your own practice at home; plus, there are plenty of simple, quick exercises and routines you can fit into a busy schedule pretty much anywhere, meaning Pilates truly can become part of your life. So, if you want a healthier, better-looking body, and a calmer mind to boot, get reading and practising now! I know I will be.

Katy Louise Evans
Editor of *Bodyfit* magazine (www.bodyfitmagazine.co.uk)

Introduction

If you're interested in keeping your body as strong and supple as possible, and your mind open and relaxed, then congratulations on opening this book on Pilates. Unlike many other forms of exercise, Pilates straddles the gap between the mind and body, which means it's ideal for toning your body, while also calming your mind.

This book will show you not just how to perform the many exercises involved in helping to strengthen your body, but how the movements and breathing can help to connect your mind and body. The goal of Pilates is to fuse the body and mind so, without thinking, your body uses the greatest mechanical advantage to achieve optimal balance, strength and health.

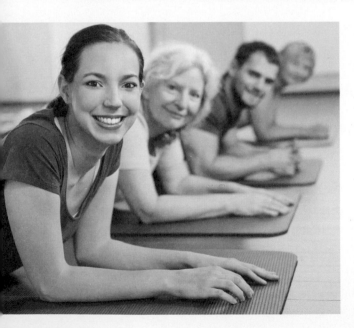

The Popularity of Pilates

Newsweek magazine reported that 5,000 people did Pilates 10 years ago; now five million in the US alone are participating in regular classes. So it must be working! In the UK, it's extremely popular, with several stand-alone Pilates foundations established, which have led to a new direction in Pilates.

The Benefits Of Pilates

There are numerous health benefits of Pilates. Weight loss, lowered stress levels, increased flexibility and reduced risk of osteoporosis are just some of the many benefits you'll find when you incorporate Pilates into your fitness regime.

Getting Acquainted with Pilates

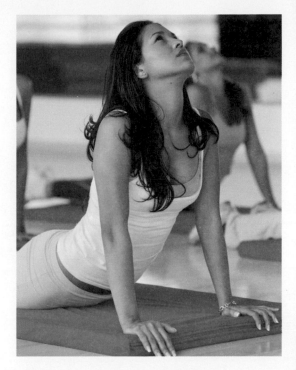

Before you begin Pilates, it's important to have an understanding of the beginnings of Pilates, how and why it started and its purpose. We'll look at the history of Joseph Pilates, the main principles of Pilates and the variations of Pilates teachings.

Although we believe that Pilates can be comfortably performed at home, attending classes is also beneficial, so we've given you a rundown of the various types of class you can attend. And not just for you, but your whole family too, at various stages in their lives.

Part of doing Pilates is understanding your body and how it works. Take the time to read about your body's structure and how it is utilized in the exercises. Your pelvis, spine, lungs and muscles are all integral to every movement, so understand their function to help you become stronger and leaner.

The Core and the Lungs

It is important to know about your 'core' and why this needs to be stabilized and acknowledged before embarking on an exercise (*see* page 18). It is also important to learn how to 'activate your pelvic floor' (*see* page 44).

Once you understand the core, learn about the lungs and the correct way to breathe – the Pilates way. This is the basis of all Pilates movements, without which you'll find that you'll tire easily and your movements won't flow. As you'll discover, learning how to breathe the Pilates way will enable you to perform the exercises correctly, as well as to hold certain moves for longer, which allows your muscles to stretch and relax.

Getting Moving

Basic Pilates movements are simple to do and easy to follow, but still, take as long as you need to do them. There's no rush! You'll find after completing one round of these movements your body will already feel more alive and flexible. These movements can be, and should be, done every day and always before you move on to the harder and more intense exercises.

Early on in the exercises chapter, you'll learn about stability – why it's so important, not just for your posture, but also for your overall structural health. Good stability means that as you get older you'll be less likely to suffer from falls and joint pain. Doing the stability exercises as many times as you can every week will help you to lay down the foundations of a strong body. These exercises provide the basics of your Pilates movements.

Basic Mat Exercises

After the stability exercises, we move on to the mat movements (pages 80–115). Ideally, use a Pilates mat, which is slightly thicker than a typical yoga or exercise mat. Read the instructions carefully and fully before you attempt each exercise. The mat movements are designed to help relieve any pain from your lower back, while building up your core abdominal strength.

Basic Standing Exercises

Your posture is, along with your breathing and pelvic floor, a vital part of effective Pilates practice. The standing exercises (pages 66–79) will show you how to correct your posture, while helping you to strengthen your abdominals and thighs and relax your shoulders. The beauty of these movements is that they can be done anywhere, at any time (within reason!). Perform these in front of a mirror if you can, as this will help you to check your posture, especially to help you confirm that you're not swaying your back, which can lead to back pain.

Good posture brings enormous health benefits: it can affect your overall health, your breath, your immune system and your energy levels. Maintaining good posture, not only when you're standing but also when you're sitting, lying down, driving or exercising, goes a long way to supporting good health.

The Next Level

You can progress on to these movements (pages 116–63) once you have perfected the exercises in the first few chapters and feel comfortable performing them without having to refer to the instructions too often. These are slightly more advanced, and you may not be able to complete the recommended number on your first attempt. Don't worry; completing just one exercise correctly is more beneficial than five half-hearted attempts. As your body becomes stronger and more attuned to the Pilates postures, you'll be able to build up the number of repetitions.

The Ultimate Level

Once you've become familiar with the previous exercises, you'll be itching to move on to a greater challenge. These movements (pages 164–87) will take time and practice – don't be discouraged if it takes you many, many attempts to master them. It's worth it though, as you'll be rewarded with a longer, stronger and leaner Pilates body.

Stretching and Cool Down

Take the time to stretch your body. Stretching will prepare your body for exercise, as well as getting you mentally ready for your session. All workouts need to end with a warm down, to allow the muscles to unwind and relax. Always make time to stretch and relax your body before getting on with the rest of your day.

Exercises with Props

Additional equipment is now used in Pilates classes, in many cases to increase the stretch or effort required to complete a move. You'll read more about props and their uses in this chapter, along with step-by-step exercises using all the props used in today's Pilates classes.

Routines for You

Whether you have 15 minutes or half an hour, there's a routine that'll suit your emotional and physical needs.

When to Do the Exercises

Ideally, you should try to incorporate Pilates into your everyday routine. Even if you only have five minutes to spare, there are several moves you can perform which will set you up for the day. Try to do a few of these morning and night to help prepare for and to undo the stresses and strains of the day. For starters, try introducing the Daily Maintenance sequence into your regular fitness routine (pages 238–50).

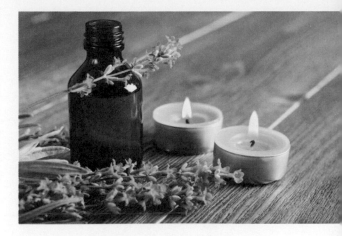

Make sure that you have the correct equipment and space necessary to perform the exercises correctly. If you prefer, put some music on (something with regular beats can help you count your breathing) and you can even burn some essential oils (such as grapefruit in the morning to motivate you, or lavender in the evening to relax you) to help set the mood.

To Help Cure What Ails You

We've also introduced movements that are specifically designed for certain conditions and ailments. You can follow these routines as part of a rehabilitation programme (such as To Strengthen Abdominals on pages 242–43). These movements have been designed with specific benefits in mind and can be done morning or night, with or without accessories.

Whether you manage to do Pilates every day or once or twice in a busy week, make sure that you set aside the time to perform the exercises properly and correctly. Pilates is a way of life that requires its own space and time, but, once you've committed to it and begun the journey, you'll never look back.

Did You Know?

One study found that after six months of Pilates, women reported feeling more satisfied with themselves and their life in general.

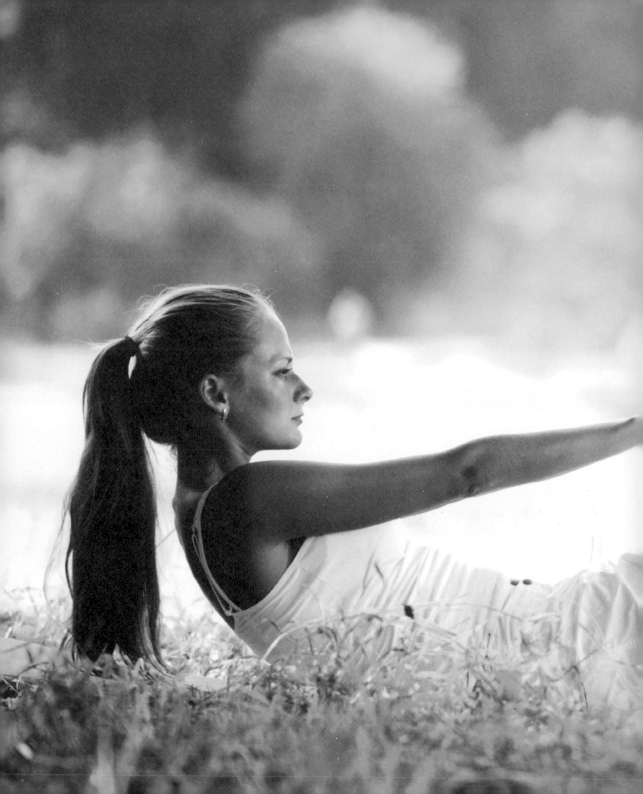

Pilates Basics

What Is Pilates?

Even though you've picked up this book, you may still be unclear on what Pilates actually is and does. To give it an official definition, 'Pilates is a form of exercise, developed by Joseph Pilates, which emphasizes the balanced development of the body through core strength, flexibility and awareness, in order to support efficient, graceful movement.'

What is Core Strength?

Core strength is the foundation of Pilates exercise. The core muscles are the deep, internal muscles of the abdomen and back. When the core muscles are strong and doing their job, as they are trained to do in Pilates, they work in tandem with the more superficial muscles of the trunk to support the spine and movement.

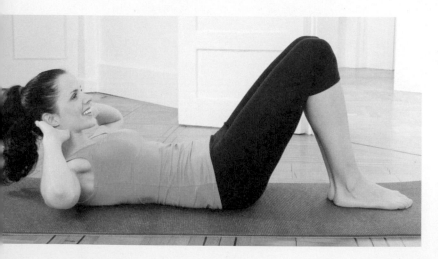

As you develop your core strength, you develop stability throughout your entire torso. This is one of the ways Pilates helps people overcome back pain. As the trunk is properly stabilized, pressure on the back is relieved and the body is able to move freely and efficiently.

How is Pilates Different from Other Forms of Exercise?

Pilates is all about working and strengthening the entire body. This absolute focus on your body helps your mind to relax and remove all extraneous thoughts from your mind. Joseph Pilates also believed that his form of Pilates, Contrology, helped to improve cognitive function.

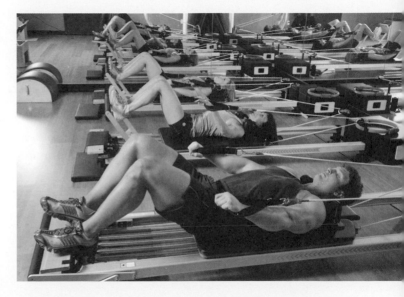

Plus, the main focus of Pilates is to help prevent injury, as well as to rehabilitate any injuries you may currently have. For instance, many ballet dancers use Pilates to help balance their workout, and rugby and football players have introduced Pilates into their fitness regime, while swimmers, cyclists and runners also incorporate Pilates into their training programmes to help enhance their performance.

Core strength and torso stability, along with the six Pilates principles (see pages 22–23), set the Pilates method apart from many other types of exercise. For instance, lifting weights can put strain on your arms or legs without including the rest of the body in the workout. Think about when you do a biceps curl: all you're doing is moving your arm – no other body part is involved. This is fine as an isolated event, but overall, for optimum health, your entire body should be involved in every movement, since that's how we are built to function. Even running or swimming can seem like all arms and legs, with either a floppy or overly tense core. Ultimately, those who really succeed at their sport learn to use their core muscles and, in Pilates, this integrative approach is learnt from the beginning.

The History Of Pilates

During the early twentieth century, Pilates movement founder Joseph Pilates said of the movements he had designed, 'In 10 sessions, you will feel the difference. In 20, you will see the difference. And in 30, you'll be on your way to having a whole new body.'

He was right. Pilates, a form of exercise favoured by millions of people worldwide and championed by celebrities such as Jennifer Aniston, Gwyneth Paltrow and Madonna, can give you a whole new postural structure and even increase your bone-mass composition.

'I must be right. Never an aspirin. Never injured a day in my life. The whole country, the whole world, should be doing my exercises. They'd be happier.'
Joseph Hubertus Pilates, 1965, aged 86

The Introduction of Pilates

Did You Know?

Regular workouts can lead to an increase in relaxation, control of mind and decreased stress.

While Pilates may seem relatively new to the masses, it was introduced almost 100 years ago by Joseph (Joe) Pilates, initially called 'Contrology'. As a boy, Joe suffered from various ailments, including rickets, rheumatic fever and asthma. Despite or perhaps because of this, he became extremely interested in health and fitness as he grew older, learning how to strengthen his body. During this journey, he trained as a body builder, gymnast and boxer.

After moving from Germany to New York, he set up a boxing studio, which just so happened to be next door to a ballet studio. He found that many ballet dancers consulted him to help their various injuries, and reported an improvement in their lower-back and abdominal strength. These new students also found that they were less likely to be injured in their dance after incorporating Pilates movements into their routines.

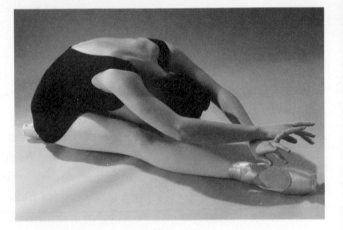

The Continuation Of Pilates

Joe sadly died in 1967, but his work was continued by many of his students and trainers, known as the Pilates Elders. While his teachings have been adapted over the years, the basics and foundation of Joe's beliefs remain the same.

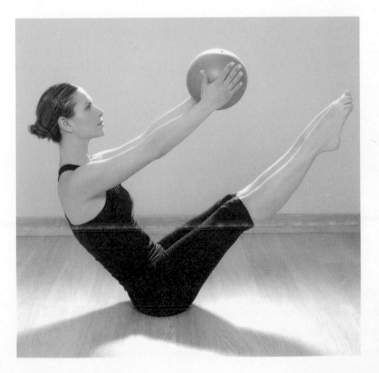

The Main Principles

In Joseph Pilates' book, *Return To Life Through Contrology*, he defined Pilates as a way to unify the body, mind and spirit. He believed that in order to completely embrace the Pilates method, something much more than mastering a set of physical movements, it was important to fully understand the six principles underpinning Pilates. By integrating these principles into your movements, he believed it was the way to achieve balance, grace and fluidity of movement.

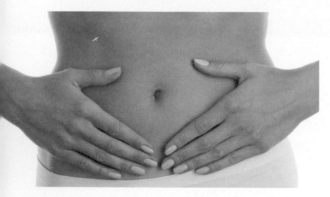

Centring

This focuses on the 'powerhouse', which is the area between the lower ribs and pubic bone. This is the basis of all Pilates exercises. A strong core or centre will help to relieve lower-back pain, hip and joint aches and improve your posture. Read more about your core on page 44.

Concentration

By focusing completely on the movement you are performing, you'll achieve better and longer-lasting results. This can be done by imagining the strengthening of your muscle or limb each time you perform a move. A workout completed with such concentration – a form of meditation – will also give your mind a break from everyday worries and distractions.

Control

Each Pilates move is completed with absolute control, and each body part has its own role to play. This may feel difficult at first, as your body is bound to struggle and wobble a bit until you build your stability, but control will come with practice.

Precision

With each Pilates move, it's important to put your hands, feet and pelvis exactly where instructed, to ensure that the movement is completed correctly. This allows your core area to fully engage so that, when you perform an exercise, your body is achieving its optimum potential.

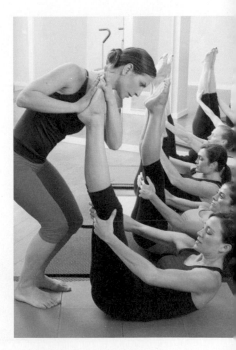

Breath

Joseph Pilates emphasized full and deep breathing co-ordinated with the movements. See page 47 for further explanation.

Flow

Even though Pilates movements are not joined together as in yoga, they still have their own grace. Thinking about gracefully moving into each exercise is a good way to introduce flow. This flow also lends itself to a more calming workout.

These principles are fundamental. They will help you to understand how Pilates works to unify mind and body and, in particular regard to the breath, will actually make the movements easier.

Classical Versus Modern

The original Pilates, referred to as Classical Pilates, is based on Joseph Pilates' original movements and the order he performed them. Modern Pilates, on the other hand, is an evolution of the movements as they have been adapted over the years.

The Evolution of Pilates

Over the past 60 years, we have learnt much about the spine and its ideal position, particularly in regard to 'neutral' spine. Originally, it was thought that the best way to perform Pilates movements was by keeping the spine flat on the ground. Classical Pilates will generally teach abdominal exercises in a 'posterior tilt', meaning that, when lying on one's back, the lower spine is completely pressed into the floor, creating a tuck in the pelvis.

We now know that keeping a small curvature in the lower spine is more beneficial to the body. Modern Pilates will generally teach exercises in a 'neutral pelvis', meaning that, when lying on one's back, the lower spine will have some space between the back and the floor, and the hip joints and the pubic bone will all be on one plane.

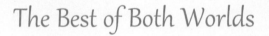
The Best of Both Worlds

The best form of
Pilates is a marriage of
the two: the classical
movements blended
with the modern
approach, with the
addition of movements
and accessories to
enhance the original
method.

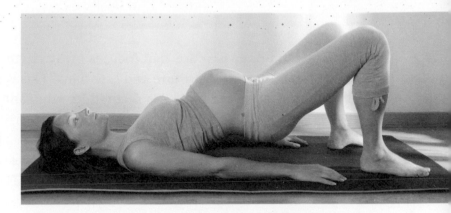

Classical Pilates will build strength and stamina, improve posture, prevent back pain, improve
flexibility and create a longer and leaner body. The developments in modern Pilates have
allowed for adaptation to individual needs and for injury rehabilitation, in addition to all the
original benefits.

The Classical Movements

The Classical Pilates movements involve seven mat moves, which flow easily from one to
another. They are listed below and you'll learn more about these in later chapters. As time has
gone by, and we have learnt more about the body, more and more movements have been
added, as well as equipment and apparatus.

- **The Hundred (page 118)**
- **Roll Up (page 124)**
- **Roll Over (page 128)**
- **Leg Circles (page 131)**
- **Rolling Like a Ball (page 133)**
- **Single Leg Stretch (page 103)**
- **Double Leg Stretch (page 109)**

The Benefits Of Pilates

Pilates is a mind-body practice that focuses on strength, core stability, flexibility, muscle control, posture and breathing. This winning combination of mind and body has secured its popularity among devotees.

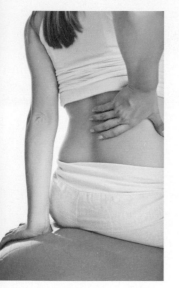

It changes your shape by educating you about how to carry yourself throughout the day, with your stomach pulled in and your shoulders relaxed and down. Even when you're not in class, you're aware of your posture and body.

Why Does Back Pain Occur?

The force of gravity acts on your spine, so poor posture will load your spine unevenly and can lead to back pain, trapped nerves and headaches. Over time, poor posture can even break down your spinal discs and cause arthritis in the spine, leading to seriously impaired mobility.

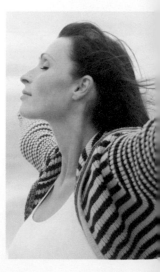

How Does Pilates Help?

Correctly performing Pilates is, as mentioned earlier, all about stabilizing the core. You do this by pulling your belly button back towards your spine, while simultaneously using your peripheral elements (arms and legs) to support you.

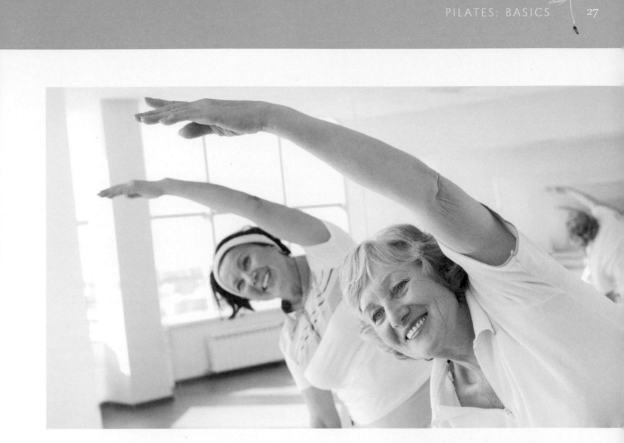

This act of stabilization is very important for those with lower-back pain or the more elderly, to improve bone density in the hips and spine. Worldwide, millions of people are affected by fragile and brittle bones – osteoporosis – which can lead to a higher risk of fractures. Pilates helps to decrease the risk of osteoporosis, as you can improve bone mass by using muscles attached to a particular site. As osteoporosis is caused by a reduction in bone mass, which leads to brittle bones, doing Pilates is a must for all women. However, if you have osteoporosis, do check with your Instructor on the possibility of certain movements, particularly mat ones, which may exacerbate your condition.

Pilates movements focus on the skeletal structure and the muscles attached to the spine and pelvis, in particular the deeper ones that lie under the surface muscles. As you become stronger, your skeletal structure becomes healthier. Pilates activates the deep postural muscles, which in turn reduces pressure on your lower back, preventing or alleviating back pain. It's thought that, worldwide, back pain costs the workplace billions of dollars every year in lost employee days, so it's worth spending time strengthening your back.

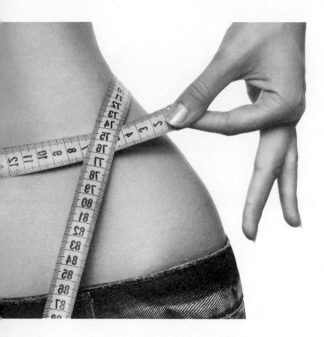

Pilates and Weight Loss

A 2011 study conducted in Turkey followed 58 obese women who attended one-hour Pilates classes four times a week for eight weeks, and found their hip-to-waist measurements and flexibility had improved. However, this is probably because their lifestyles were largely sedentary prior to taking up regular exercise, and so any exercise would have made a difference. No amount of Pilates will help give you a six-pack or reduce the amount of fat around your belly, but it can and will inspire you to begin and maintain a healthier lifestyle.

For the Mind

Unlike many other exercises, whereby your mind is free to wander while your body performs the same tasks over and over again (such as running, walking or cycling), Pilates engages the entire focus of your mind to perform the tasks. This intense focus means that you're less likely to be worrying about external issues, which allows your mind a rest from your usual daily stresses. And, as your mind is focusing on what your body is doing, there is a much better connection between the two.

Checklist

☐ **For your health**, Pilates is one of the most important choices you can make for your mind and body, as it's a great all-rounder.

☐ **Flexibility** can help to reduce lower-back pain and make you feel stronger, younger and more supple.

☐ **Strengthening** your body can help to reduce ill health and, the more muscle mass you have, the lower your body fat content. It's a win-win.

☐ **Joseph Pilates** was the founder of Pilates, which he introduced to New York during the 1960s. It is now practised worldwide.

☐ **The many different** types of Pilates all stem from the same belief: a strong body equals a strong mind.

☐ **Whether** you're looking to increase your flexibility, find stress relief, fix a bad back or address other skeletal issues, Pilates can help with most of your health concerns.

☐ **The core** is the, well, core of Pilates. This is where all movement and energy comes from.

☐ **Classical versus modern** Pilates is a long-standing debate, but it is thought that a blend of the original doctrine and the modern approach is optimal.

☐ **The many benefits** of Pilates include a more youthful body, elongated, lean muscles and a more relaxed, focused mind.

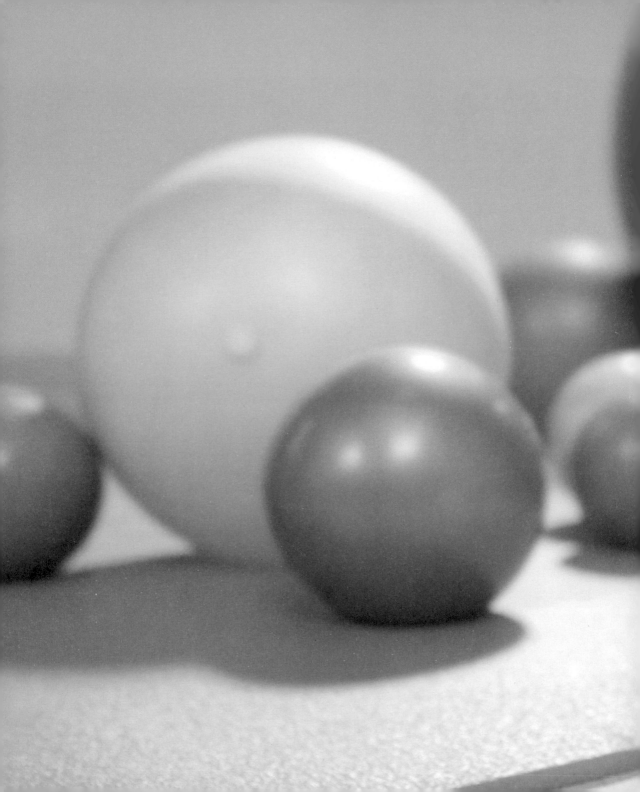

Getting Ready

Who Can Do Pilates?

Pilates is for everybody, regardless of your age, fitness level or flexibility. It's relatively simple to do, once you've learnt the basics, and you don't even need to attend classes in order to do some moves. All you really need is the motivation, some instruction or knowledge of the exercises and a mat. However, if you have specific health issues, you might want to look into specifically tailored classes.

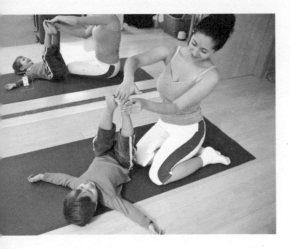

Pilates for Children

Ideally, children should do 60 minutes of exercise every day. However, more and more children are becoming increasingly sedentary, leading to a rise in obesity in the young. While this recommended 60 minutes should ideally be aerobic activity (running, swimming, cycling and so on), Pilates can be a useful complementary activity, as some movements, such as the hundred, increase the heart rate, while others focus on calming the mind and stretching the body.

Pilates and Teenagers

Pre-teens and teens can also benefit from Pilates. One study found that a group of 11-year-old girls who took part in a four-week Pilates class five times a week, lost weight and reported high enjoyment. As always, enjoyment of exercise is the primary reason for continuing the activity.

Pre- and Post-Natal Pilates

Pilates can help to reduce the lower-back pain associated with pregnancy. The stomach and pelvic floor muscles are put under increasing strain as the baby grows, which can cause pain and discomfort. At the same time, the hormone relaxin is making the tough tissues (ligaments) that connect your bones more pliable. This can lead to instability in the body. As Pilates uses the deepest layer of the stomach muscles, the movements help to stabilize the back and pelvis.

Post pregnancy, helping the stomach muscles to knit together again and strengthening the pelvic floor are of huge benefit. The stretching and relaxation side of a Pilates class are also ideal for any sleep-deprived, exhausted mothers.

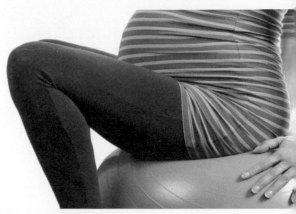

Over 50s

Joseph Pilates said: 'Physical fitness is the first requisite of happiness. In order to achieve happiness, it is imperative to gain mastery of your body. If at the age of 30 you are stiff and out of shape, you are old. If at 60 you are supple and strong, then you are young.' Pilates exercises are not only ideal for those over 50 who wish to regain health and mobility, but also for those who wish to guard against falls and osteoporosis.

When Pilates is not for You

If you have extreme back problems or health issues, it's important to check with your GP or Pilates instructor before commencing Pilates. A modified version of exercises may be available, or other forms of stretching could be recommended.

Classes

When Joseph Pilates taught his method, he did one-on-one consultations only, which allowed him to focus all his attention on his student. Nowadays, many Pilates classes, especially those in gyms, can have up to 30 or so participants.

Types of Classes

You can arrange one-on-one teaching, but it tends to be pricey, although it is worth the initial investment if you can afford it. This will enable you to pick up the fundamentals of the movements and find out what your common mistakes are. As a good compromise, Pilates schools tend to run classes of around six to eight. This is a good number to allow the teacher to give each student some personal attention.

Classical Classes

These involve mat work, although you can use accessories such as weights, lumber pillows or Swiss balls. These classes are ideal as part of your overall fitness regime.

Machine Versus Mat Work

Stretching and strengthening your body doesn't involve only poses on a mat. There are now Pilates reformer machines, accessories such as magic circles (see page 37) and vibration machines. The best idea is to do mat and machine work in a supervised class where you'll use both mat and props to help strengthen your core. Reformer machines act as an aid to help you get into position or to perform the move, while mat work uses your own bodyweight to perform the moves and as resistance.

Do You Need A Class?

It's perhaps a little unusual for a book like this to direct you to a class, but when it comes to Pilates, yes, you should initially at least go to a few classes. This will help you learn the foundations of breathing and to locate your core, as well as identify any mistakes before they become habits. A good teacher will help show you what to watch out for. This way, when it comes to using this book at home, you'll know what you need to keep an eye on.

Finding A Class

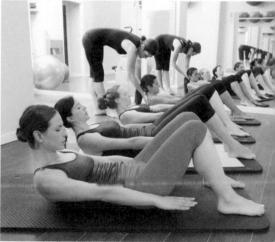

Finding the perfect Pilates class, like any other exercise class, tends to depend on the individual. One teacher's way of teaching may not be to your particular taste, or may just not suit your needs. Ideally, the best classes are found through word of mouth or recommendation. Obviously you can start your search on the internet (see page 253).

Check Out the Teacher

As anybody can do a six-week course and open a Pilates studio, it's important to check out the qualifications of your teacher. Ideally, they should be Pilates mat and reformer trained, a qualification that takes around two years to attain. If you're in doubt, or just want to find the best teacher near you, contact the national body in your country.

The Art Of Self-Practice

While it's great to attend a Pilates class, whether it's for an introduction, for further knowledge or even just the social aspect, one of the great advantages of Pilates is it can be practised anywhere. Once you have a mat and a bit of space, you can get started, at any time, in any place, for as long as you like.

Three Key Points

When Should I Practise?

Ideally, you should do a Pilates session first thing in the morning. This has the benefit of helping warm up your muscles and stabilize them for the day ahead. A lovely stretch will help you to start the day the right way. If you can, set aside at least 30 minutes a day for your routine.

Should I Eat Before My Class/Routine?

Researchers are still debating about whether we should eat before or after exercising. If you find you get to the middle of your session and all you're thinking about is your breakfast, then have a banana or some oatcakes before you begin. Keep a bottle of filtered water to hand at all times to keep hydrated.

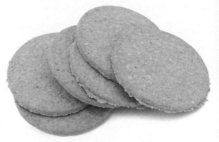

How to Make it a Habit

As with anything, in particular exercise, it can be difficult to find the time to fit in your practice. If mornings are too busy, then take a look at your evenings. Can you miss (or record) that television programme and do 30 minutes then? With 24 hours in a day, we should all be able to find time for 30 minutes of exercise.

Pilates Essentials

While there are specific Pilates outfits you can buy, there's really no need to splash your cash. A pair of stretchy leggings, sports bra (if applicable) and top are all you need. Wardrobe sorted, there are various pieces of Pilates equipment you can invest in if you decide to make Pilates part of your everyday life.

What Kit Do I Need?

Invest in a thick Pilates mat – they are available at most sports stores, Pilates schools or over the Internet. Look for one that's a little thicker than a standard fitness mat, to help support your body.

Some other useful bits of kit include:

- **Pillow:** These can be slightly curved or just one inch thick, and are used to support your neck during some exercises. You can substitute with a folded towel or blanket.

- **Magic circle:** Propped between your knees or ankles, this is a relatively new Pilates accessory which can enhance your workout. They can take some getting used to, but you will feel the difference when using them – especially in your inner thighs.

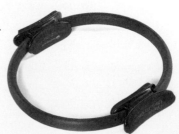

- **Stretch band:** Like a magic circle, using a stretch or resistance band can help increase the intensity of your exercise.

Leg weights: Very similar to Velcro-attached weights used in other exercise classes, these help you to tone and sculpt your muscles.

Hand weights: The hand weights used for Pilates are very light – less than 1kg. If you don't have any available, you can use a can of beans or filled water bottle.

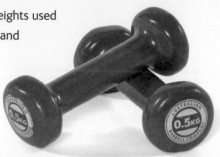

Music: Create a relaxing ambience by playing some music while you work out. It can help you focus on your breathing and prevent your mind from wandering.

Water: As with all exercise, you should sip room-temperature water while working out to prevent tiredness and dehydration.

Blanket: If you have time to finish your workout with a meditation, cover yourself with a blanket to keep your muscles warm.

Pilates exercise balls: Looking like an overinflated beach ball, and sometimes called a Swiss ball, the big balls are a wonderful way to perform some moves if you aren't able to use the mat, or for some specific ball-based movements. Some people also use their Swiss balls to sit on at their desks, or as part of their stretching and exercise regime at the end of the day. The small ball is a wonderful way to massage sore, tired muscles and provide support for some movements. It's important to release some air from the ball, otherwise your neck may be propped up too high.

Checklist

- ☐ **Everybody** can do Pilates, no matter your age or fitness ability. There's a class to suit everyone.

- ☐ **Children** can benefit from Pilates, as it encourages their natural flexibility while helping them to focus their minds and take time to learn relaxation techniques.

- ☐ **There are many schools** of Pilates. There's no right or wrong school, as they're all based on the teachings of Joseph Pilates. It's about finding which is best for you.

- ☐ **Home practice** is one habit you should develop. You don't need much to practise at home – just some space and a thick exercise mat.

- ☐ **Just 15 minutes** of Pilates every day can be of huge benefit to your body and mind.

- ☐ **Props** can be used for some exercises, such as yoga bands, a magic circle, foam roller or Swiss ball.

- ☐ **Introducing props** into your workout can give it an extra dimension and challenge, as well as preventing you from becoming bored or too used to your workout.

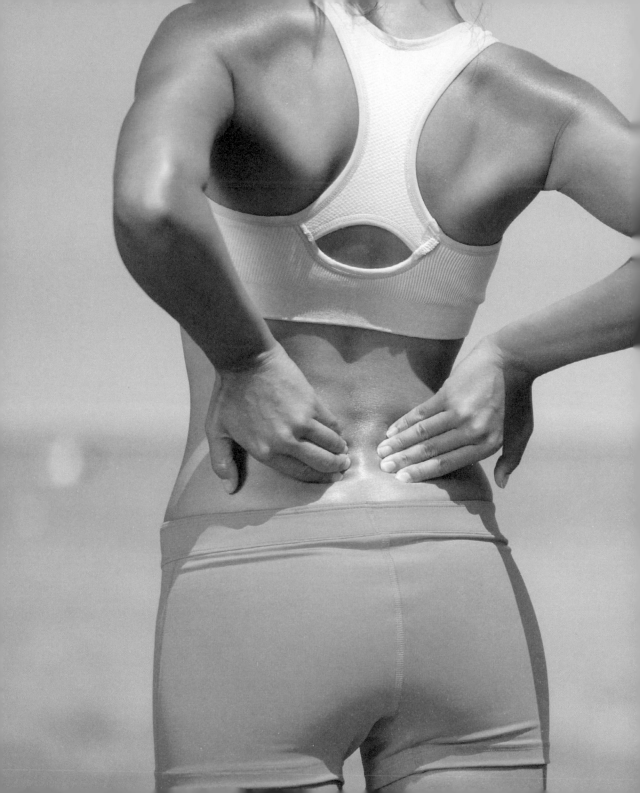

The
Pilates
Body

The Anatomy Of Pilates

When you first go to a Pilates class, or indeed, as you read through the exercises in this book, you'll come across various words, such as core, activation, pelvic floor and Pilates breath. These terms relate to the way you use your body throughout each movement.

The Core

The core applies to the band of muscles that sits under your ribcage and either side of your spine. This area is important when it comes to your overall body strength, as every movement you make originates from here. Hence, when this area is unstable, or weak from underuse, instability occurs, which can lead to injury and imbalance. The core is made up of more than just your abdominals and back. There's a whole layer of muscles under your torso, including your pelvis and your back.

Your core muscles include:

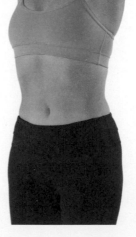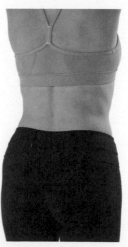

- **Multifidus:** Deep spinal muscles that run from the neck to the centre bone of the chest.

- **External obliques:** Muscles on the side of the waist that attach at the lower ribs, pelvis and abdominal fascia (see right).

✎ **Internal obliques:** Internal waist muscles or abdominal muscles that attach at the lower ribs, rectus sheath, pelvis and thoracolumbar fascia.

✎ **Transversus abdominis:** Abdominal muscles that attach at the lower ribs, pelvis, thoracolumbar fascia and rectus sheath.

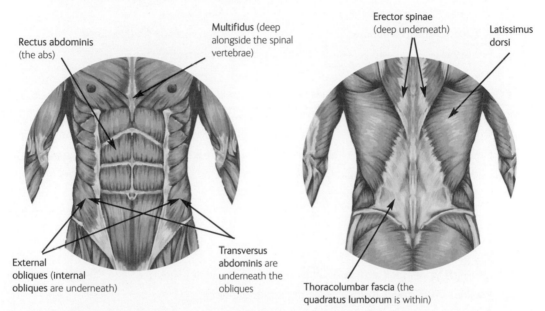

Rectus abdominis (the abs)

Multifidus (deep alongside the spinal vertebrae)

Erector spinae (deep underneath)

Latissimus dorsi

External obliques (internal obliques are underneath)

Transversus abdominis are underneath the obliques

Thoracolumbar fascia (the quadratus lumborum is within)

✎ **Rectus abdominis:** A pair of muscles that run vertically on the front wall of the abdomen, generally referred to as 'abs.' This is the primary abdominal muscle that attaches to the lower sternum and the front of the pubic bone.

✎ **Abdominal fascia:** These connective tissues join the obliques and rectus abdominis to the pectoral muscles.

✎ **Latissimus dorsi:** A pair of dorsal muscles also known as 'lats'. This muscle is the largest spinal stabilizer and helps perform all the pulling motions through the arms.

- **Erector spinae:** This paired bundle of muscles and tendons runs the length of the back.

The core muscles all work together to support the lumbar spine (the lower part of the back).

- **Quadratus lumborum:** This muscle stabilizes the spine while allowing flexibility.

- **Thoracolumbar fascia:** Think of this as a net. It connects and holds the lats, glutes, internal obliques and transverse abdominals and supports the spine.

It's not important to memorize all these muscles, but it is important to realize just how complicated your core is, and why it's imperative to keep it stabilized and strong. Knowing how and when your core is centred is one of the first skills you'll learn in Pilates. It's not just a matter of pulling your belly button in as much as possible. Neither is it keeping your hips and stomach muscles as rigid as possible (which would just lead to back problems).

How to Activate Your Core

1. **Lie with your back and feet flat** on the mat and your knees bent at a 90-degree angle.
2. **Flatten your lower back** by pressing it into the floor.
3. **Arch your back** slightly by lifting your hips.
4. **After a while, achieving this position** will come naturally, but until then, practise this movement before beginning your Pilates workout to ensure you are at 'neutral'.

How to Activate Your Pelvic Floor

The easiest way to activate your pelvic floor, or to 'turn the muscles on', is to imagine that you have to do a wee but need to either hold it in or stop halfway. It may sound a bit strange, but practising with this in mind can help you become more aware of the 'activation' you need to awaken your pelvic muscles.

The Spine

Our spine is the most important part of our skeletal system, affecting our health, posture and mobility. Pilates focuses on finding the neutral position of the spine before beginning an exercise. This is because your core needs to remain stable whilst moving other parts of the body. In other exercises, you'll move your spine and pelvis.

The Spine: A Biology Lesson

Our posture is the first thing people notice about us. Bad posture can make you look tired, lacking in confidence and even give the appearance of weight that's not really there. But upright, good posture can make all the difference to your appearance and inner health. You'll look (and feel) more confident, taller and yes, even slimmer.

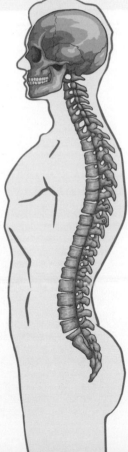

We are all born with a natural S-shaped spine, but over time, due to skeletal issues, lack of exercise and age, the curve of the spine changes, which may place undue stress on the ligaments, muscles and intervertebral discs. Over time, pain sets in.

Pilates helps to rediscover the natural S-curve in the spine, as well as creating space between the vertebrae. You will notice within a short time of beginning Pilates that you'll walk taller, have less lower-back pain, be more flexible and be able to move between sitting and standing positions more easily.

Muscles

You use almost every muscle in your body when performing a Pilates movement – whether it's the abdominal muscles, pelvic floor muscles, neck and shoulder muscles or leg muscles.

More conventional or traditional workouts are weight bearing and tend to build short, bulky muscles – the type most prone to injury. Pilates elongates and strengthens, improving muscle elasticity and joint mobility. A body with balanced strength and flexibility is less likely to be injured.

The Role of Muscles in Pilates

While the focus of Pilates is mainly on your spine and pelvis, your muscles also play an important part in your movements. The idea is to utilize all – spine, pelvis and muscles – whenever you're doing an exercise. A balanced workout will include these equally, mobilizing your spine and utilizing your muscles in the front and back of your body to strengthen them.

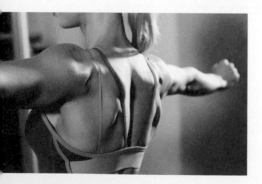

Challenging the Muscles

Certain movements will challenge your muscles more than others. These are:

- **Curl Ups (page 91)**
- **Oblique Curl Ups (page 92)**
- **The Hundred (page 118)**
- **The Teaser (page 180)**

The Lungs: Breathing

We all know how to breathe, right? Wrong! Many of us breathe incorrectly, that is, taking short, shallow breaths. This does very little to relax or oxygenate the body. In fact, it can create more stress to the system and our muscles.

How To Breathe

Breathing is an integral part of a Pilates movement – it helps you to relax the body, stretch further and focus the mind. It's important to create a rhythm with your breathing rather than a forced movement, as this can interrupt the flow of the Pilates breath that we are aiming to achieve.

How To Find Your Lungs

Sit on a mat and wrap a stretch band around the lower part of your ribs, crossing over at the front. Hold the opposite ends of the band and pull tightly. Breathe in, and focus on the back and sides of your ribcage – this is where your lungs are located.

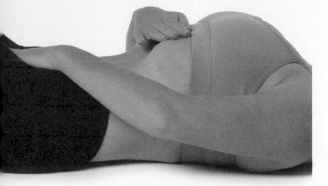

Top Tip

**Don't hold or force your breath.
If you miss your breathing cue,
just begin the exercise again.
You shouldn't have to think about
what you're doing.**

Imagine a balloon gently filling with air –
this is how your breath expands your lungs
and ribcage. With each breath, keep your
shoulders relaxed, breathe in through your
nose and out through your mouth.

Or, lie on a mat with your knees bent and
place your right hand at the bottom of your
rib cage, and your left hand on your pelvis.
Breathe in and notice the way your ribs lift
upwards and outwards. Your pelvis should
remain neutral. Continue to practice this
way of breathing until it becomes natural.

Top Tip

**Take a couple of breaths before starting a more difficult move.
It will mentally prepare you for the stretch.**

Checklist

☐ **Posture** is an important part of our health we can focus on each day – it will help you feel more confident, breathe more easily, deal with stress and prevent back and neck pain.

☐ **A neutral spine** is important, as it allows some space between the back and the floor when lying on one's back. A neutral spine makes exercises easier to perform and prevents pain.

☐ **Osteoporosis** is a condition that causes low bone density and brittle bones, common amongst the elderly. Practising Pilates improves bone density by increasing bone mass.

☐ **Postural muscles** are the muscle groups around the spine and hips. Pilates develops the postural muscles located deep below the surface, resulting in a strong skeletal structure, crucial in preventing lower-back pain.

☐ **Our lungs** are important to us, as they not only help us breathe, but are our powerhouse and source of our energy through oxygen, so take the time to breathe properly.

☐ **Breathe in** whenever it's time to prepare for a movement, as it will help you to relax and focus your mind. **Breathe out** whenever it's time to make your move – it'll help you activate your abdominals and stabilize your pelvis.

☐ **Relaxation** is your main aim whenever you're doing Pilates, so make sure that you enjoy your session.

☐ **Weight loss** can be positive side effect of Pilates, as it is proven to encourage a healthy lifestyle and thus reduce weight.

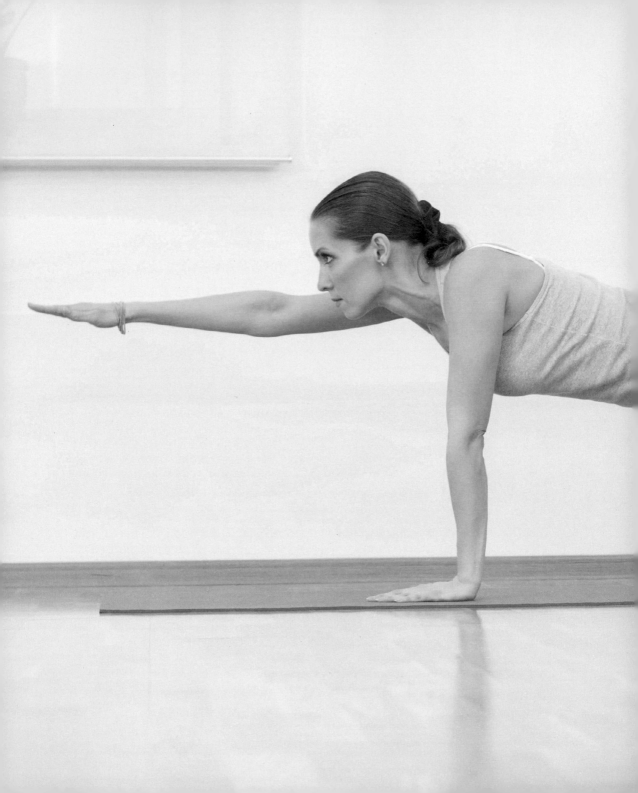

The Exercises

Getting Started

Pilates takes a softly-softly approach to beginning your workout. It's important to familiarize yourself with these movements so that in time you do them without having to refer to the book.

The Exercises

The exercises are designed to flow from easy to slightly harder. As you work through the exercises, you'll move from the basic, introductory movements to the harder, more advanced ones. Take your time to learn these. If the recommendation is to complete up to five repetitions, and you find at first you can't do these, perform one or two well and work your way up as you become stronger and more flexible.

Introduction to Your Stability

These are the foundation exercises, which provide the basics for the more advanced movements you'll learn as you become more practised.

Basic Standing Exercises

These will help you to align and correct your posture.

Basic Mat Exercises

Learn to keep your spine and pelvis neutral.

The Next Level

As you become more experienced and flexible, move on to these more difficult positions.

The Ultimate Level

Once you graduate to this level, you'll be able to automatically mobilize your spine and pelvis. The earlier chapters will also be part of your usual routine.

Stretching and Cool Down

Use these invaluable exercises to prepare your muscles for activity and, importantly, help return them to resting after your workout.

Exercises with Props

This following chapter shows how introducing Pilates props into your exercise routine can help you advance your movement and also confirm your posture.

Routines for You

This chapter provides some tailored routines. Find a 15- or 30-minute routine that's designed for your needs.

Introduction To Your Stability

Your stability is the most useful and important thing you can achieve in Pilates, and it will serve you well in life. It will help to alleviate back pain, ill health, headaches and abdominal issues. With stability, you'll be able to control your movements, which means you'll be less likely to inflict any injury on your joints or muscles.

The exercises on the following pages will help you to find your stability and perform them without moving your spine or pelvis. If you move your spine or pelvis during a movement, this can lead to instability and pain.

Why You Should Do These Exercises Daily

Learning and improving your stability by doing these exercises as often as you can will ensure that it becomes part of your everyday life, not just when you're exercising.

Ideally, do these exercises every day. By doing so, you'll find you'll begin to stand taller, sleep better and complain of less lower-back and hip pain.

What to Remember

While stability is important, keep in mind that there is a difference between 'stability' and 'rigidity'. Keeping your pelvis and spine still and firm is different to holding your pelvis and spine fixed into position. Keeping too rigid will stop any particular flow of movement. If anything, holding yourself too firmly will create tension in the muscles.

Before You Begin

Practise getting your body into neutral position by focusing on your abdominals, pelvis and spine (see Setting Up on the following page). When this position becomes natural to you and you can breathe naturally without thinking about it, begin the stability exercises and introduce them to your daily routine.

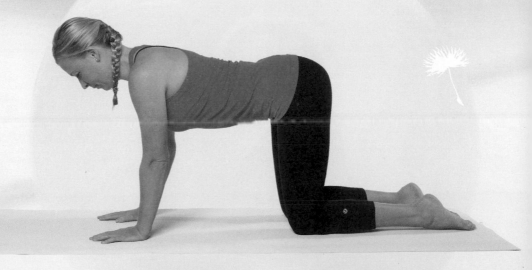

Setting Up and Starting Position

This is the starting pose for many mat exercises. Practise it daily to help you find your neutral pelvic and spine position. You can also return to this position whenever you need a breather.

1 **Lie on your mat** with your legs bent, feet hip-width apart, arms resting by your sides, palms upwards.

2 **Turn off your muscles** all over by breathing in and out deeply, relaxing your body as much as possible. Check that your spine is relaxed and your pelvis is in neutral.

3 **Gently draw** in your pelvic floor. You should be able to feel that your lower abdominals become slightly firm.

Top Tip

Do this movement as often as possible, even in between movements, to ensure your position is correct.

4 **Check** that your neck and shoulders are relaxed and that you are breathing evenly and deeply.

5 **Remain here** for around one minute, or longer if you prefer.

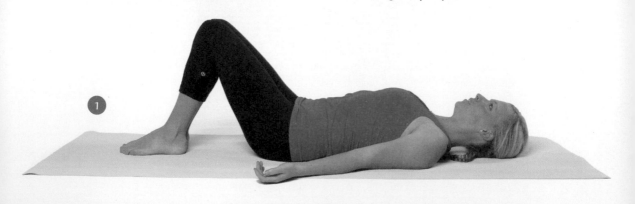

Cat Stretch

A lovely extension for warming up your back and awakening the abdominal muscles. Try doing this every morning and evening to release any tensions in your body.

1 **Kneel on your mat**, keeping your back flat, your arms directly below your shoulders and your knees under your hips. As you inhale, gently reach the middle of your back towards the ceiling, lowering your head and tucking your tail bone under.

2 **As you exhale**, reverse the curve in the spine by sinking the spine to the floor and holding your head up and bottom out. Ensure that your shoulders are away from your ears. Draw in your pelvic floor and lower stomach.

3 Repeat **six** times.

Top Tip

When you return to neutral, keep your back flat; don't be tempted to let your muscles go or your spine drop towards the floor.

Extended Cat Stretch

If you want to achieve further mobility in the spine, then add this wonderful back stretch into your routine. It not only stretches your spine, but also opens your hips, relieving back pain and increasing flexibility.

1 **Repeat steps** 1 and 2 of cat stretch.

2 **Return to neutral and inhale.** On the exhalation, lower yourself to the left of the mat, reaching your arms in front of you, palms flat on the floor. Feel the stretch all the way to your fingertips. Your bottom will be resting on your lower calves and ankles, toes pointing to the back of the mat.

3 **Stay here for five breaths**, feeling your muscles relax further with each exhalation.

4 **Slowly move** your upper body to the right, slowly feeling your way with your

fingertips across the mat, until you reach the right side of the mat. Stay here for **five** breaths.

5 **Return to the centre**, with your arms straight out in front of you, palms facing downwards. Exhale and return to step 1.

Top Tip

This movement is ideal for those who sit at a desk all day, to counterbalance a slumped posture.

2

Knee Openings

Practise your stability between your pelvis and spine, while stretching your legs from the hip joints. This is the starting point for all the knee-opening movements.

1 **Lie on your back** on the mat, with your spine relaxed and stretched from top to bottom. Your knees should be bent, with your feet flat on the ground. Make sure that your pelvic floor is activated (*see* page 44).

2 **Breathe out** and slowly separate and lower your knees towards the floor. Check that your back hasn't arched – your spine, pelvis and hips need to remain neutral. Allow your feet to roll on to their outer edges.

3 **Slowly bring your knees** back together on the inhalation, keeping your abdominals strong and firm.

4 Repeat **five** times, keeping your hips neutral.

Top Tip

A good way to check that you haven't moved is to pay attention to your buttocks. You should be able to feel that they are evenly placed on the floor.

2

Single Knee Openings

Find your stable position with this exercise. This movement helps you to find neutral each time you return to the start.

1 **Lie on your back**, knees bent, hands facing upwards. Your spine should be evenly placed on the mat. Inhale, pulling your belly button back towards your spine and tightening your pelvic muscles.

2 **Place your hands** on your hips if you need to check that they are stable.

3 **Exhale and allow** your left knee to slowly open. Your left foot will slowly roll on to its side. Take this movement as slowly and carefully as you need to, making sure that your hips remain

stable. Open your knee as far as you can without creating strain or pain in your lower back.

4 **Return** to the starting position. Repeat on the right side. Do the move **five** times on each side.

Top Tip

If you experience pain at any time, stop immediately. Begin the exercise again, taking the movement more slowly and with less of an opening.

1

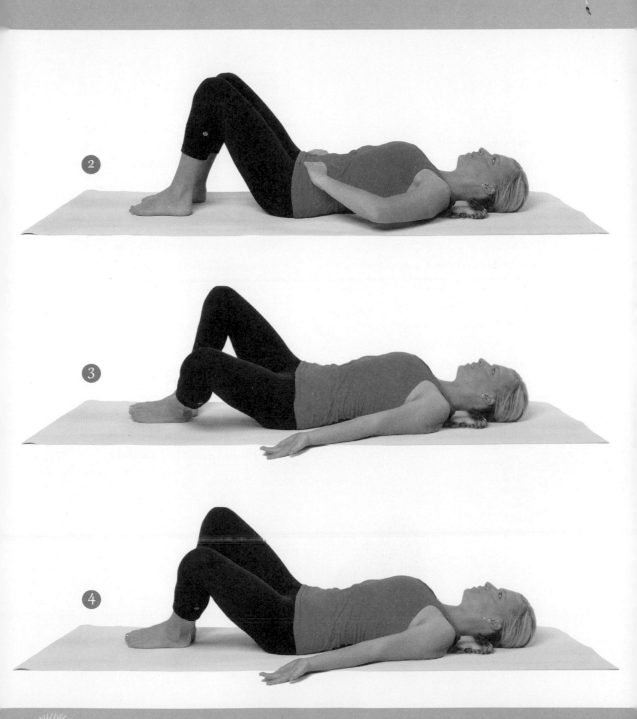

Leg Slides

This move will help you to warm up your hips and lower back and strengthen your core stability. It's also good practice for learning to complete smooth movements with your limbs.

1   **Lie flat** on your back, knees bent. Check that your pelvis is activated (*see* page 44). Place your hands on your hips if you need to ensure that they are balanced and neutral.

2   **Breathe out** and engage your pelvic floor and abdominals as you slide your left heel away from your body, keeping your leg in line with your hip. Breathe in and return your leg to the bent position.

3   **Repeat the movement** with the right leg, ensuring that your pelvis stays stable and in neutral position.

4   Repeat **10** times on each side.

Top Tip

Make sure that you don't arch your back. Keep your spine neutral throughout the movement.

Imprinting

As the name suggests, you feel as if you are 'imprinting' your body on to the mat, ensuring that your spine is long and lean and your hips are neutral.

1   **Lie on your mat**, knees bent, feeling as though your body is sinking into the floor. Your pelvis should be activated (*see* page 44).

2   **Slowly lift your pelvis** off the floor so that you achieve a slight curve and space in your lower back. Hold for the count of three and return to the start.

3   **Repeat this movement** as often as you like in order to feel natural in this pose.

Top Tip

Imprinting is one of the most basic movements, but one of the most important. Practise this move whenever you need some rejuvenation.

Arm Openings

After spending a day at your desk, relax your shoulders and neck with this exercise that helps to align your head, neck and upper body.

1 **Lie on the mat** on your back with your knees bent and your arms reaching up towards the ceiling, palms facing towards each other. Make sure that your shoulders are even and they haven't risen towards your ears. Activate your pelvic floor (*see* page 44) and breathe in.

2 **As you exhale**, bring your arms down to reach out on either side of your body, palms facing upwards. Your movements should be slow and fluid.

3 **Return** to the first position and repeat **six** times.

Top Tip

Make sure that you don't lift your hips or lower back from the floor, as this will place unnecessary strain on your lower back.

Overhead Arms

Open up your ribcage and abdominals with this lovely stretch. It also takes away any tension from your lower back.

1   **Lie on your back** with your knees bent. Your spine should be neutral and your hips even. Activate your pelvic floor (*see* page 44) and breathe in and out. Your arms should be resting on either side of you, palms facing downwards.

2   **Place your shoulder blades** so that your upper body is slightly lifted from the ground. Slowly raise your arms up and over, lowering both arms to the floor behind you, resting your fingertips on to the floor. Keep your shoulders stable, and make sure that they don't move up towards your ears.

3   **Breathe in** and, as you exhale, return to the starting position.

Top Tip

Don't let your ribs lift or arch your lower back. It's important to retain a neutral spine throughout this movement.

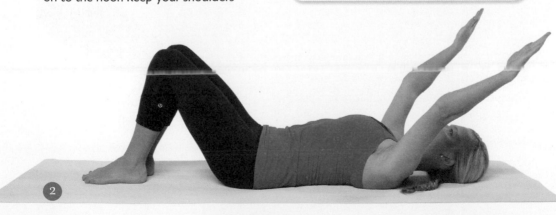

Basic Standing Exercises

The following movements will help to improve your overall posture, confidence and everyday stability. By practising these movements as often as you can (ideally every day, or at least three days a week), you'll learn awareness of good posture, how to relax your mind and how to release tension, particularly in your neck, chest and shoulders.

Why Standing Exercises Are Good for You

Standing exercises are part of your overall workout, balancing the mat work with the upright poses. They also provide a link between the Pilates mat work and everyday movement. This way, correct posture and alignment become a natural part of your life.

Each of the standing postures is designed to help you fully mobilize your spine and the muscles in the front and back of your body. Some exercises are slightly more advanced in order to build greater spinal movement and flexibility.

Before You Begin

Finding your symmetry is an important step when beginning standing exercises. Ideally, look in the mirror to check your posture and ensure the following:

- **Your head is directly above your shoulders.**

- **Your shoulders are low and equal.**

- **Your palms are facing towards your thighs.**

- **Your hips are level and not pushed forwards or backwards.**

- **Your legs are straight and firm, but not locked at the knees.**

- **Check that your ears are in line with your shoulders, that your head isn't pushed forwards or too far back.**

- **Your stomach is pulled in slightly, without too much effort.**

- **Your spine has its natural curve.**

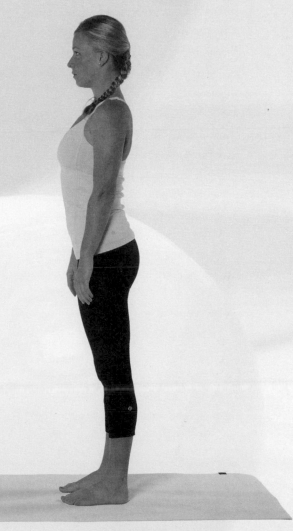

Floating Arms

This is a good exercise to do before and after a routine, as it warms you up and helps to cool muscles down. If you suffer from sore neck and shoulders or associated headaches, this can help to reduce pain and relax your muscles.

1   **Stand in the middle** of your mat, feet evenly placed hip-width apart, arms loosely by your side, neck and shoulders relaxed.

2   **Draw** your abdominal muscles inwards. You should feel your torso lengthen and your posture straighten.

3   **Breathe in**, lengthening your spine by pulling your torso slightly upwards.

4   **Breathe out**, activating your stomach muscles as your raise your arms outwards, slowly reaching up towards

4

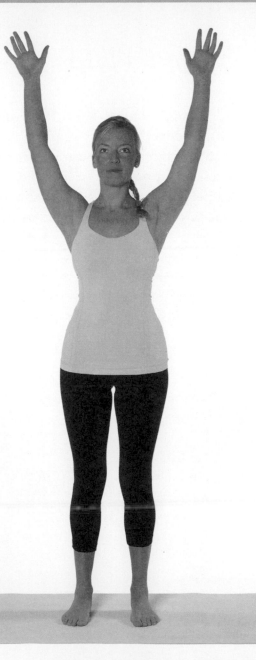

the sides of the room. Keep your arms and hands soft and make sure that your shoulders haven't risen up towards your ears.

5 **To warm up**, you can repeat this halfway movement **five** times, to practise the flow of the steps.

6 **To continue on**, slightly rise up on to your toes, simultaneously lifting your arms above your head. Your stomach muscles should be engaged. Make sure your bottom hasn't stuck out behind you as you lift your arms. If you feel that you're going to lose your balance, fix your eyes on a spot a few metres in front of you: this will help you maintain your equilibrium.

7 **Breathe out** and slowly lower your heels to the floor and your arms by your sides.

8 Repeat **five** times.

6

Tennis Ball Rising

It's as important to strengthen your legs as it is your abs, to ensure fluid movements and stability. This is a simple move which can be done using a wall or chair as support. It can be done at your desk to help strengthen and lengthen your quads, as well as stretch out your spine.

1 **Stand on your mat** with your feet just slightly apart. Tuck your bottom under and activate your pelvic floor (see page 44).

2 **Place a tennis ball** between your ankles, just slightly under the anklebones. The ball shouldn't be touching the floor.

3 **For balance**, place your hand against a chair.

2

Top Tip

Imagine that there is a rope attached to your head, pulling you upwards. This will help you keep your posture upright, so that you don't lean forwards or backwards, which can place undue pressure on your spine and hips.

4   **Activate your core** (see page 44) and breathe in. Breathe out and rise up on to the balls of your feet. Be careful not to lean forwards or backwards. Take it slowly. Make sure that you're balanced evenly on your toes and that your feet haven't rolled outwards.

5   **Use your pelvic muscles** and legs to keep the ball firmly between your ankles.

6   **Breathe in** and lower your heels back to the mat.

7   Repeat **10** times.

Standing On One Leg

Maintaining balance and building stability are the main foundations of Pilates. This move helps you to find your centre, whilst strengthening your ankles, feet and thighs.

1 **Stand** with your feet hip-width apart, hands loosely by your sides. Look straight ahead, neck and shoulders loose and relaxed.

2 **Activate your core**, and breathe in. Check that your posture is correct, your spine long and your pelvic floor activated.

3 **Breathe out** and, very slowly, shift your weight on to your left foot, without moving your hips or pelvis. Make sure that your toes don't scrunch up or your foot rolls outwards.

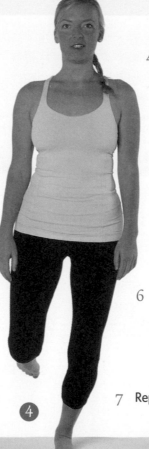

4

4 **Bring your right knee** slowly upwards towards your body.

5 **When your right knee** is at a 90-degree angle to your body, hold for the count of three, breathing evenly. Make sure that you haven't swayed slightly to the left.

6 **Breathe out**, slowly returning your foot to the mat and distributing your weight evenly over both feet.

7 Repeat **five** times on each leg.

Pilates Squats

A deceptively easy-looking exercise, which works your thigh muscles and challenges your stability.

1   **Stand on your mat**, feet almost touching. Straighten your body so that you're in the correct starting position, looking straight ahead, pelvic floor activated, shoulders and neck relaxed.

2   **Breathe in**, and slowly lower your body towards the floor by slightly bending your knees. Don't allow your upper body to slump, keep your spine long and upright.

3   **At the same time**, slowly lift your arms in front of you, palms facing downwards, keeping them shoulder-width apart.

4   **Slowly lower yourself** further, trying not to slump forwards. Your arms should rise at the same time, until at shoulder height. Turn your palms slowly to face each other, without lifting your shoulders.

5   **Breathe out** and return to the starting position.

6   Repeat **10** times.

Wrist Circles

We use our hands quite a bit in Pilates to hold our body weight, or to fully stretch from top to toe. This exercise will help to reduce stiffness or tension in the wrist and forearm.

1 **Stand on your mat** with your feet slightly apart and your hands straight out in front of you, palms facing downwards.

2 **Feel the stretch** in your arm as you extend the feeling through to your fingertips. Make sure that you don't move your shoulders forwards as you stretch.

3 **Breathe in** and, as you exhale, slowly rotate your hand, in a full circular motion as follows.

4 **Lift your fingers** up to the ceiling, then to the side, before lowering down towards the floor. Return to the starting position with hands straight out. Repeat with both hands in clockwise and anti-clockwise rotations.

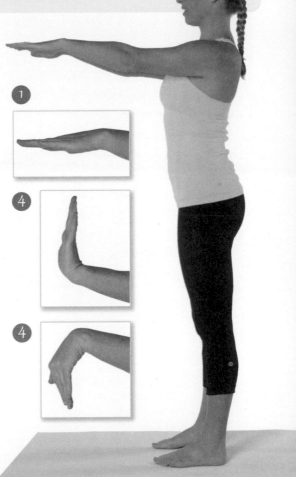

Dumb Waiter

This exercise gets its name as it looks as though you're carrying a tray! However, it's a great move to open your chest area and increase mobility in the upper arms.

1   **Stand on your mat**, feet parallel and hip-width apart.

2   **Bend your elbows**, so that your arms are at a 90-degree angle, your upper arms are close to your side and your lower arms are reaching forwards. Turn your palms upwards.

3   **Activate your pelvic muscles**, breathe in and, keeping your hips and shoulders still, open your arms from the shoulder joints, reaching to either side as far as you comfortably can.

4   **Breathe out** and return to the starting position.

5   Repeat **10** times.

Top Tip

Check that you are using your shoulder joints to perform the movement, not the elbow. You'll notice a squeezing in your side if your elbows are the lead motivator.

Cocktails Anyone?

This is a lovely stretch for your lower back, while enforcing the stability of your pelvic area. Take the move slowly and only turn as far as you feel comfortable.

1   **Starting from step 2** of the Dumb Waiter (*see* page 75), breathe in and slowly turn to the left. Turn from your waist and keep your hips stable. This may take some practising, so just perform a small movement initially.

2   **Hold here** and breathe out. Check that your thighs and knees are facing forwards and your hips haven't tilted.

3   **Return to the starting position** on an inhalation. Hold here for the count of three, breathing regularly. Breathe in and slowly turn to your right, again making sure that your hips remain stable.

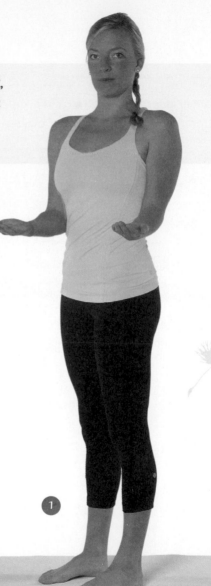

1

Top Tip

If your arms and shoulders begin to ache, return to the starting position and check that you're not holding your arms too tightly against your sides. Your shoulders should be loose and relaxed, with your head held upright. Check that your core is activated and your spine elongated – this will take any tension away from your shoulders and neck.

4   **Hold and breathe out** and return to the starting position.

5   Repeat **five** times on each side.

Roll Down

Slowly unravel any tension in your spine, while strengthening the muscles in your back and hips. Your bottom and hips also benefit from this move.

1   **Stand with your feet** firmly planted on your mat, hands loosely by your sides. Your spine should be tall and strong, abdominals and pelvic floor activated.

2   **Breathe in** and, very slowly, tip your head forwards, making sure not to slump your shoulders forwards or push your bottom out.

3   **Continue** breathing regularly (deep breaths in and out) as you curl downwards, stretching your spine.

Top Tip

If you're just beginning, it may be a good idea to practise this move against a wall to help you feel the sensation of slowly rolling your spine, vertebra by vertebra.

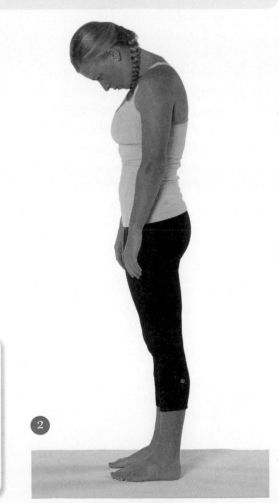

2

4 **Halfway down**, allow your head to relax forwards, your ribcage and breastbone to soften. Then continue your downward trajectory as your arms fall forwards.

5 **Stop** when you feel your hips move or contract.

6 **Allow yourself** to relax here for a few breaths before slowly returning to the starting position.

7 **Take it slowly**, don't rush any movement and imagine that you're stacking your vertebrae one on top of another as you return to the starting position.

Advanced Moves

If you want to introduce a further stretch, after step 6 slowly allow your body to drift to the left, stretching the right side of your body. Repeat on the other side, remembering to keep your hips stable.

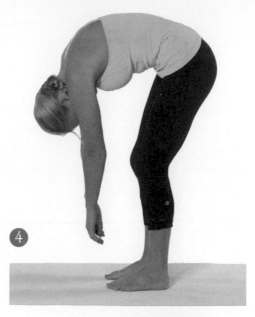

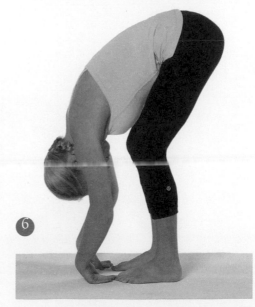

Basic Mat Exercises

**Now it's time to relax on the floor. Although that's a bit misleading...
You may be lying on the floor, but you'll be working hard. One of the main
focuses of mat work is to achieve and maintain stability and mobility in
the pelvis and spine, while achieving control and flexibility of your body.**

The Benefits of Mat Work

Lying on your mat will allow you to practise core stability. By doing these exercises as often as
possible, you'll be able to find your core stability quickly and easily. The following movements
will stretch your spine and create flexibility. By engaging your arms and legs, you'll also build up
your core strength.

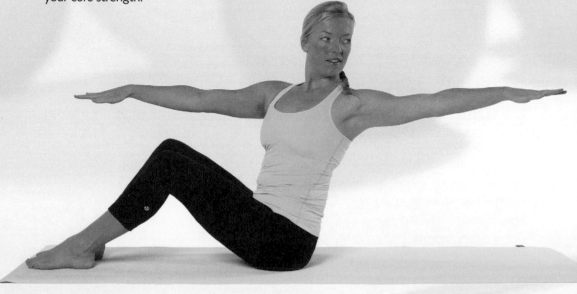

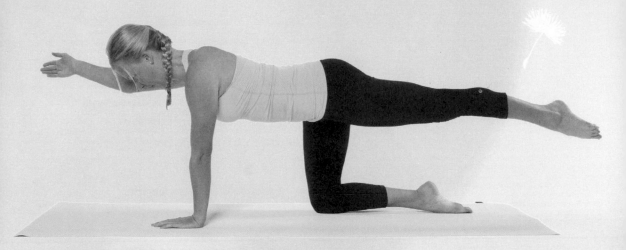

How Often You Should Do Mat Work

Ideally, do mat work every day, either morning or evening. All you need is your mat and some space to perform the movements. Some movements, such as curl ups, imprinting and rest position are ideal to do at the end of each day to relax and unwind your mind and body.

What You'll Need

Other than a Pilates mat, which should be a little thicker than a typical exercise mat, you may need some support under your head, particularly if you have lower-back or neck pain. A small pillow (as seen here for example) can be a useful neck support in some movements.

Shoulder Drops

If your head and neck ache and crack after a day at the desk (especially if you prop your phone between your neck and your shoulder), then this is an ideal movement for you, and it can be done at any time of the day.

1   **Lie on your mat** with your knees bent, your arms by your sides, palms facing upwards. Lift both your arms up so that they're shoulder-width apart, palms facing each other.

2   **Breathe in** and reach your left arm up towards the ceiling. You should be able to feel your left shoulder blade lift away from the mat.

3   **Breathe out** and bring your arm back down until you feel your shoulder blade back on the mat.

Top Tip

Make sure that your elbows aren't locked out; keep them slightly soft.

4   Repeat up to **10** times.

5   **Repeat** with the opposite arm.

Arm Circles

Sitting at a desk or just daily life can cause stress and tension around your neck and shoulders. This movement helps to release this through the shoulder blades, while creating stability in the spine.

1   **Lie on your mat**, knees bent, your arms by your sides, palms facing upwards.

2   **Breathe in**, making sure that your spine and pelvis are in neutral.

3   **Breathe out**, lifting your arms directly above your shoulders, hands reaching towards the ceiling, palms facing inwards.

4   **Continue** the movement, by lowering them over your head towards the mat. Make sure you're not lifting your shoulders or lower back during this movement.

Top Tip

Avoid locking your elbows when your arms are behind your head, otherwise your shoulders will rise upwards, undoing your good work.

5   **Breathe in** as you bring your arms in a circle out to the sides and down towards your body.

6   **Return your arms** to the sides, palms facing the ceiling.

7   Repeat up to **five** times, then again in the reverse direction.

Pelvic Clocks

This movement helps you become aware of the difference between neutral position and moving your pelvis and spine in a controlled manner. Knowing this can help you alleviate back pain and improve your Pilates performance.

1   **Lie on your mat** with your knees bent and your feet flat on the floor. Make sure that your legs are parallel and your ankles, knees and hips are all in one line.

2   **Check** that you are in neutral spine position.

3   **Breathe in** and out, relaxing your shoulders and neck.

4   **Breathe in**, allowing your ribs to expand.

5   **The idea of this exercise** is to imagine a clock lying on your lower abdomen, upside down as you view it. You move your pelvis to various points on the clock: 12 o'clock (belly button); six o'clock (top of your pubic bone); three o'clock (left hip bone); nine o'clock (right hip bone).

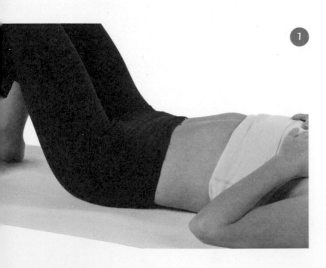

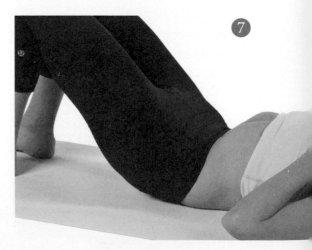

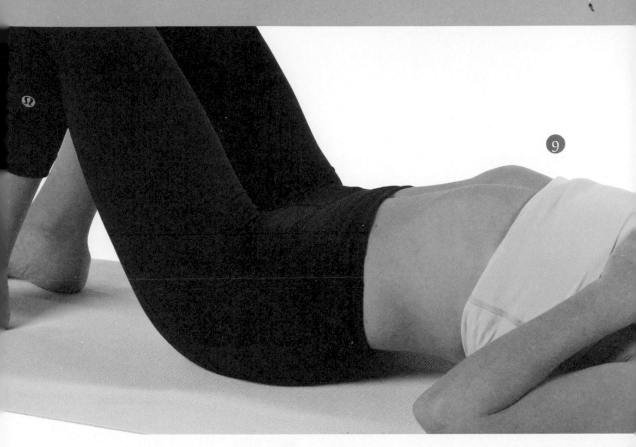

6   **Breathe out and focus** on your abdominal muscles. These need to be engaged to move your pelvis.

7   **Inhale and exhale**, engaging your abdominal muscles to bring your belly button towards your spine, so that your spine is flat on the floor.

8   **Inhale**, then rotate your abs to rotate your clock round to three o'clock.

9   **Continue breathing out** and move around to six o'clock, before moving on to nine o'clock.

10 **Return to 12 o'clock**. Repeat three times in this direction, before repeating **three** times in the opposite direction.

Pelvic Rolls

These are ideal to do before and after your exercises, as they warm up the pelvic area and reinforce your stability.

1. **Lie in the starting position** with your pelvis and spine in neutral.

2. **Breathe in** and expand your ribcage, lengthening through your spine.

3. **Tilt your pelvis** slightly backwards, taking care not to overdo it. You should feel your spine imprinting itself on the floor.

4. **Slowly tilt your pelvis** the other way, stopping any time your lower back hurts.

5. **Switch** between these two positions, enjoying the slight massage on your lower back.

6. **Repeat** as many times as you like.

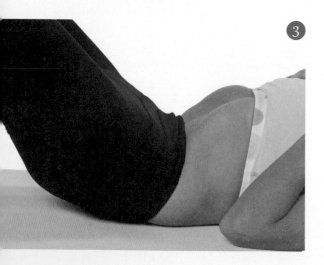

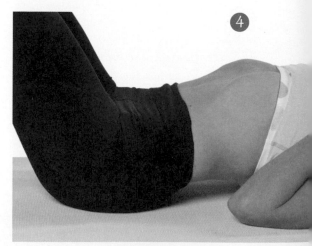

Bridge

This movement helps to strengthen your glutes as well as lengthen your lower back and spine.

1   **Lie on your mat** with your knees bent, arms by your sides.

2   **Breathe in** and prepare to keep your back stable as you exhale, then focus on lifting from the hips and thighs.

3   **You should be able to feel your thighs** and insides of your legs working hard. If they start to wobble, stop and begin again, but don't lift as high this time.

4   **Continue rolling** up the spine to an elevated shoulder plank. You may wish to hold this pose and then return to the starting position. As you get stronger, then continue on to steps 5–6.

5   **Inhale**, then, as you breathe out, lift your left leg up towards the ceiling at a 45-degree angle, so that your thighs are still parallel, your toes pointed. **Hold here**, then return your foot to the floor, before lowering your bottom back to the mat.

6   Repeat up to **five** times with your left leg and again with the right leg.

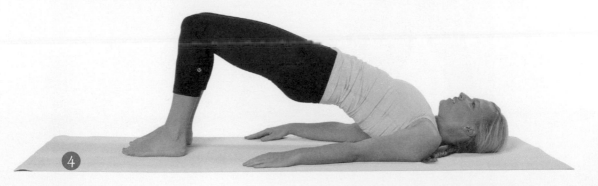

Windows

This is a wonderful way to open up your chest area and get the blood flowing in your arms.

1   **Lie on your mat** in the relaxation position, arms reaching up to the ceiling, keeping your arms above your shoulders, palms facing inwards.

2   **Lower your elbows** to the mat, keeping them bent. They should be just lower than your shoulders. Don't worry if your hands or forearms don't touch the mat, this flexibility will come in time.

3   **Breathe out** and lower your forearms, reaching out towards the back of your mat so that your fingertips have lowered on to the mat.

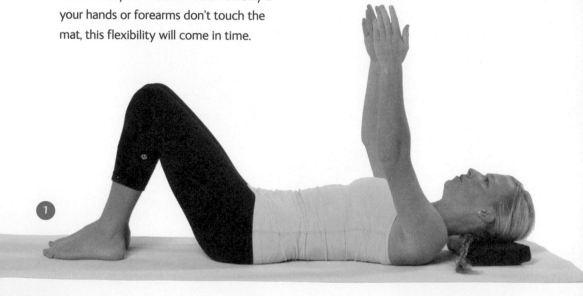

Continue to stretch your arms out, so that they're reaching to the back of the mat.

4   **Breathe in** and return your arms to above your chest, back to the starting position.

5   Repeat up to **ten** times.

Top Tip

Make sure that your shoulder blades don't ride upwards as you reach backwards. By stretching as far as comfortable without moving your shoulder blades, you'll keep your position stable.

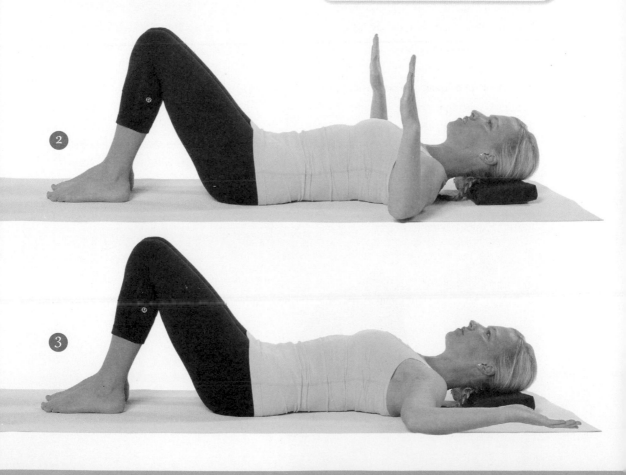

Knee Circles

This move looks simple, but is an effective way to isolate your hips from your thighbone. This movement is particularly good if you suffer from lower-back pain, or discomfort that comes from sitting for too long at your desk.

1   **Lie on your mat** with your knees bent to around 45 degrees, arms by your sides, feet flat on the mat.

3   **Focus on the lower leg** you're about to lift (in this instance, the left leg), and breathe in, then slowly lift your leg. Moving from the hip and holding the bent knee, move the knee in clockwise motions as you lift, and circle until your leg is parallel with the floor and your knee has been brought towards your hip.

4   **Repeat five times**, then circle your lower leg in an anti-clockwise direction. Then repeat on the other side.

Top Tip

Perform this move slowly, otherwise the temptation will be to lift your lower back from the floor and move your pelvis and abdominal muscles. By performing the movement slowly, you'll be able to keep your pelvic area stable.

3

Curl Ups

Also known as 'chest lifts', these look like old-fashioned stomach crunches, but done slowly, they will stabilize your spine and help you to practise keeping your pelvis firm.

1 **Lie on your back** with your knees bent, feet flat on the floor. Make sure that your legs are parallel, lined up so that your hip, knee and ankle are in one line and your toes are pointing directly away from you.

2 **Keep your shoulders down** as you bring your hands behind your head with the fingertips touching. Your hands should be supporting the base of your skull.

3 **Take a few deep breaths**. Use this time to make a little survey of your body. Be sure your body is balanced widthways. Check that your neck is relaxed and your ribs are dropped.

4 **Exhale**. Slowly pull your belly button down towards your spine and keep going, allowing your spine to lengthen out and the lower back to come down to the mat. Simultaneously tilt your chin slightly down and, with a long neck, slowly lift from the top of your head so that the top of your spine is off the mat and the bottoms of your shoulder blades are just brushing the mat.

5 Repeat **five** to **10** times.

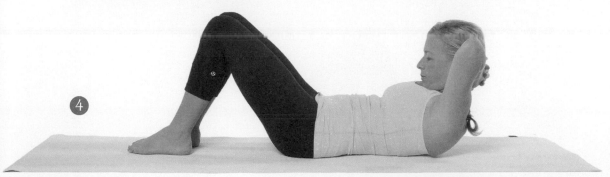

Oblique Curl Ups

These movements are a natural advancement of the curl ups, although the focus is on strengthening the abdominals and the muscles on either side of your waist.

1 **Lie on your back** with your knees bent, feet flat on the floor, pelvis and spine in neutral. Clasp your hands together behind your head, releasing your elbows wide but keeping them in your peripheral vision. Keep your shoulders relaxed and away from your ears and keep your neck long. Allow your head to be heavy in your hands.

2 **Breathe in to prepare** and lengthen your spine. Breathe out as you nod your chin towards your chest, and begin to curl your upper body off the mat.

3 **Rotate your spine** to the left, directing your breastbone towards your left hip. Feel your waist and lower abdominal muscles working. Keep your feet grounded and pelvis still – twist only from your ribs.

4 **Breathe in** wide into your ribcage and maintain the position, deepening your abdominal connection.

5 **Breathe out** and slowly release to come back to the centre. Repeat up to **10** times, and then repeat on the other side.

Hip Rolls

This challenges the abdominals and obliques, and reminds you to stabilize your pelvis and spine. It's also a wonderful way to release any tension or pain in your upper body.

1 **Lie on your mat** and bring your feet and knees together and engage your pelvic floor. Relax your shoulders and place your arms at your sides, palms facing up or down, whichever feels best for you.

2 **Breathe in to prepare** and lengthen through your spine. Engage your entire core as you begin to rotate your hips and legs to the left. The right side of your bottom and pelvis will slightly lift off from the mat – allow this to happen.

3 **Exhale** and, checking that your abdominals are still activated, bring your legs back to the starting position.

4 **Breathe in** and roll to the other side.

5 Repeat up to **five** times.

Advanced Moves

Repeat step 1, then float one knee and then the other so that your lower legs are parallel to the floor. With your knees together, slightly lower your legs to your left, keeping both arms firmly on the ground. Return to the centre and repeat on the right. Repeat up to five times.

2

Table Top

Get some well-defined abs with this pose, which helps you to create a strong and balanced centre.

1   **Kneel on your mat** with your hands directly below your shoulders and your knees below your hips. Keep your spine in neutral, with a very soft curve. Your neck should be relaxed and long, eyes focusing on the mat.

2   **Breathe in** and lengthen through the spine. Imagine that a string is pulling

your head slightly forwards. Feel the stretch through your neck and spine.

3   **Breathe out**, draw in your abdominals and stretch your right arm forwards, keeping it in line with your shoulder. Make sure that your shoulder hasn't crept up or tensed. Breathe in and bring your right arm

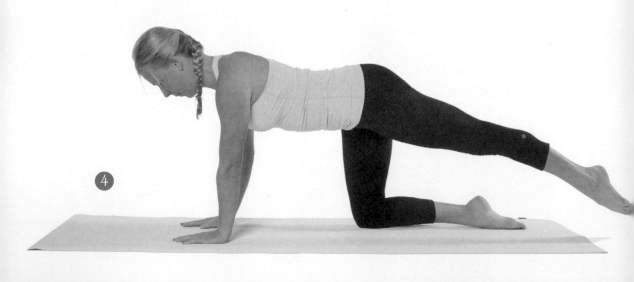

back to the ground. Repeat with the left arm.

4   **Breathe in** and lengthen your left leg behind you, keeping it slightly lower than your bottom. Your toes should be pointed.

5   **Breathe out** and return your leg to the starting position and repeat on the other side.

6   **If you have managed the above**, then you can try a more advanced move. Breathe in, concentrating on your stability. Then breathe out, sliding your

left leg backwards and lifting it up, foot pointing until it's almost in line with your hips. At the same time, lift your right arm, stretching it forwards.

7   Repeat **eight** times on each side.

Top Tip

If you wobble too much when you lift your leg, keep your toes in contact with the floor to help you balance.

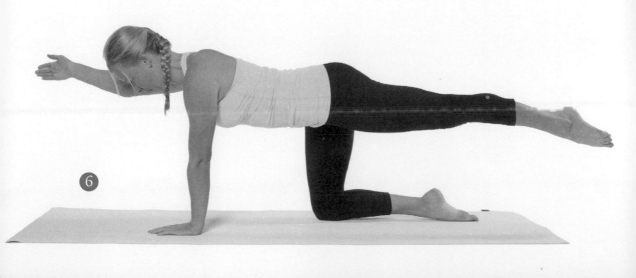

6

Diamond Press

This exercise looks very easy, but if you have sore neck and shoulder muscles, it can be difficult to achieve. Only lift as far as is comfortable.

1   **Lie on your stomach** with your legs hip-width apart and your arms bent, so that they form a diamond shape. Rest your head on your hands.

2   **Breathe in**, focusing on a strong core and stable hips and spine.

3   **Breathe out** and bring your belly button back towards your spine while slowly sliding your shoulder blades down your back. You should naturally feel an impulse to lift your head.

4   **Gently and slowly** lift your head, keeping your eyes on the mat and your arms on the floor.

5   **Stay here for one breath**, then breathe out and return to the starting position.

6   Repeat up to **10** times.

Top Tip

Avoid pressing down on your arms as you lift your head. The movement should come from your abdominals, not your arms and shoulders.

Dart

Strengthen and stabilize your back muscles, while creating a strong core.

1 **Lie on your mat**, face down, arms on either side of your body, palms facing upwards. Your toes should be pointed towards the end of your mat.

2 **Breathe in**, feeling the lengthening of your neck and spine.

3 **Breathe out**, slowly lifting your head, then your neck from the mat. Keep your eyes facing down to the mat to avoid lifting your head upwards.

4 **Breathe in** and hold this position, while lengthening as much as possible through the spine.

5 **Breathe out** and return your head to the mat.

6 Repeat up to **10** times.

Top Tip

Your feet should stay on the mat at all times. It may be tempting to lift them. If so, don't raise your head so high.

Book Opening (Sitting)

A great move to open up your chest and shoulders and to release any tension in your lower back.

1　**Sit on your mat** with your knees bent, your abdominals activated, posture upright and your arms out straight in front of you.

2　**If this places** too much pressure on your spine, sit on a cushion or a rolled-up towel. Some people prefer to perform this move sitting on a chair. Do whatever works for you.

Top Tip

Check that you're sitting evenly on your bottom throughout the movement. This will ensure that your pelvis remains stable.

3　**Breathe in**, checking your posture; you should be sitting upright.

4　**Breathe out** as you bend your left elbow back towards your body, as you turn from your waist, keeping your head in line with your arm.

5   **Breathe in** and straighten the left arm, so that it's at around 70 degrees to your body. Check that you haven't slumped forwards.

6   **Keep your arm straight** and breathe out as you return your straightened left arm back to the starting position.

7   **Repeat** on the other side, then repeat **five** times on each side.

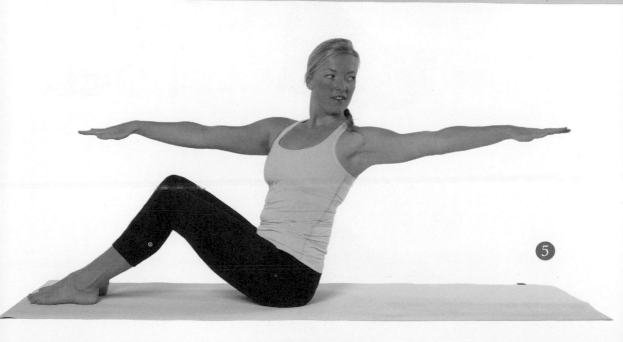

Book Opening (Lying)

Similar to the previous movement, although this movement opens up the chest, head and neck area, while stabilizing the hips and pelvis.

1 **Lie on your left side** with a small pillow under your head for support. Your knees should be bent, feet and legs on top of each other, arms stretched out in front. Your palms should be facing each other.

2 **Breathe in**, and bend your right elbow, keeping your fingertips in contact with the inside of the left arm, as you slowly lift your arm to the centre of your chest.

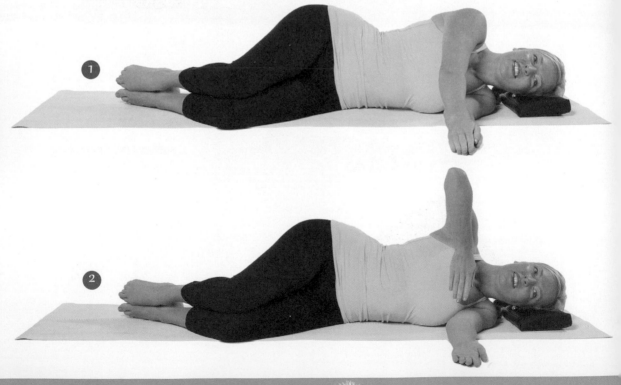

5

3   **Turn your head** towards the right, along with your shoulders and spine.

4   **Breathe out**, rotating your spine further, but not so that you cause any pain or discomfort.

5   **Breathe in** and straighten your right arm up towards the back of the mat. You should feel a wonderful opening in your chest area. Make sure that you haven't lifted your shoulders upwards.

6   **Breathe out** and rotate your spine back to neutral, as you drop slowly back on top of your left arm.

7   **Repeat** up to **five** times, then swap positions and repeat on the right side.

Top Tip

Add light hand weights to the movement. When you reach halfway, pause here before continuing to lower your arm to the ground behind you.

Arm Openings

This is a great way to open and relax the chest area, while teaching control of the torso. You can use a light handweight (no more than 1 kg) to increase the stretch.

1   **Lie on your** left side with your head resting on a small pillow.

2   **Place your arms** out in front of you, feet resting on top of each other, knees bent.

3   **Breathe in**, stabilizing your core, lifting your right arm to reach up towards the ceiling. Meanwhile, reach out with your left arm in front of you to stretch your shoulder blades.

4   **Keep your knees** and pelvis as still as possible, while softly rotating your spine towards the left, lowering your left arm down towards the mat.

5   **Breathe out** and return to the starting position.

6   **Repeat five times**, then change positions and repeat on the right side.

Top Tip

Your arm should lift naturally with the rotation of the spine. It may take a few practices before this comes naturally.

Single Leg Stretch

This strengthens the legs, as well as being a wonderful stabilizing and firming movement for the abdominals.

1 **Lie on your back** on your mat, with your knees bent, feet on the floor.

2 **Breathe in** and check that your pelvis and spine are stable and that your lower back or bottom isn't off the floor.

3 **Breathe out**, slowly lift your head, neck and upper body and legs off the floor, reaching your arms to the outsides of your lower legs or knees. You should be in a lightly curled up position.

4   **Breathe in** as you slowly lower your left leg to the mat, so that your foot is flat on the floor. Once here, slowly slide your foot along the mat until your leg is straight. Try to make sure that you don't tilt your hips or pelvis while doing so.

5   **Pull your right knee** slightly towards your torso, keeping your toes pointed on both legs.

6   **Repeat on the other leg** by slowly bringing your left leg back to your torso, while dropping your right foot to the floor. Slide your right foot out straight, keeping your toes pointed.

7   **After you have repeated** the movement on each leg five times, pull both legs towards you so that your body is curled into a ball. Gently rock your body back and forth to massage your spine.

8   **Roll your head back** to the floor and slowly lower your legs one at a time to the floor until you're back in the starting position.

Top Tip

Your legs should be moving independently from your hips and your spine. If your stomach muscles rise, then you need to restart, checking your stability before beginning again.

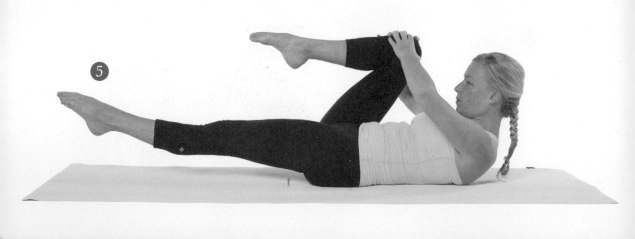

5

Oblique Single Leg Stretch

This alternate leg stretch helps you to maintain a strong core, while stretching out the oblique muscles.

1   **Lie on your back** on your mat with your knees bent, feet parallel and hip-width apart. Your spine and hips should be in neutral.

2   **Breathe in**, focusing on your abdominals, keeping them tight and firm.

3   **Breathe out**, raising your head and neck. Your hands should be lightly positioned behind your head as though you're doing a sit-up.

4   **Lift your legs** into a 90-degree angle with your body. Your stomach muscles should be firm and stable.

Top Tip

Use your abdominal muscles to lift your head, not your neck muscles (don't allow the tendons on either side of your throat to tense).

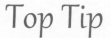

4

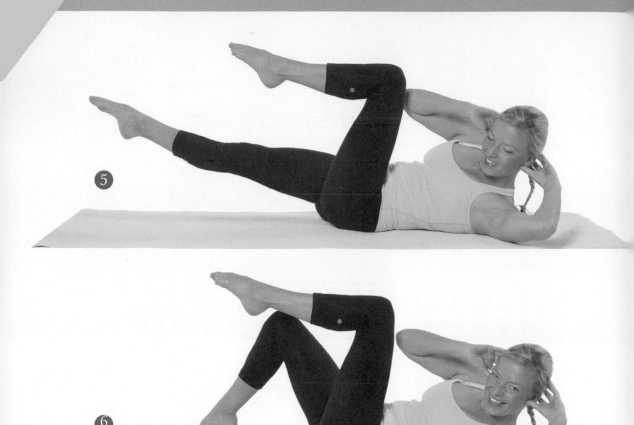

5   **Breathe in** and stretch your right leg outwards at a 45-degree angle to your body. Meanwhile, your left leg should be brought back towards your torso. Bend your right elbow towards your left knee to stretch out your shoulders.

6   **Breathe out**, inhale and swap legs, reaching to the right knee with your left elbow.

7   Repeat **five** times on each leg.

Knee Rolls

Ideal if you suffer from sore or creaky hips. This movement helps you to increase the mobility of your hip area, while emphasizing the stability of your knees and ankles.

1   **Lie on your mat** with your knees bent, feet together.

2   **Breathe in**, checking that your hips and spine are stabilized.

3   **Breathe out and s**lightly roll your knees to the right, so that your spine and feet roll together. At its furthest reach, your knees should be slightly off the floor.

1

3

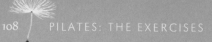

⑤

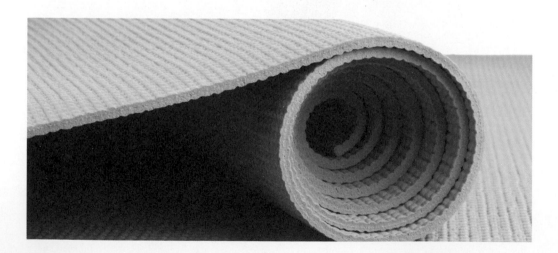

4 **Make sure** that the effort is coming from your legs, not your back or hips.

5 **Breathe in** and return to the centre before smoothly rolling to the left side.

6 **Return** to the centre and lower your knees.

7 Repeat **five** times on each side.

Top Tip

There is some movement allowed in the hip area in this movement here, otherwise your posture will be too rigid. For beginners, only roll slightly from side to side until you become used to the exercise.

Double Leg Stretch

This is a great overall stretch that strengthens the spine while challenging the abdominal muscles.

1 **Lie on your mat** with a small pillow under your head. Your hands should be palms up, arms at your sides, knees bent.

2 **Bring one leg** at a time to a 90-degree angle at the knee. At the same time, bring your head and neck up and your hands behind your head.

3 **Breathe in** and then, as you exhale, stretch your legs out, toes pointed. Check that you haven't lifted your lower back from the mat.

4 **Hold this pose for a breath**, then, as you breathe out, bring your knees back to the bent position.

5 **Continue** this routine up to **10** times.

6 **To return to starting position**, slowly lower your head back to the floor, followed by your feet. Then slide your feet back to the starting position.

3

Clam

This is a great way to open up the muscles around the hip joints. Make sure that you don't open your legs too far, as this can create stress on the hip and lower-back area.

1   **Lie on your left side** with your left arm extended above your head and in line with your body. If you find this slightly uncomfortable, place a towel or pillow between your neck and your arm.

2   **Place your right hand** on the mat in front of your body, bending your elbow to support your body.

3   **Bend your knees**, with your feet behind you.

4   **Breathe in**, stabilizing your pelvis and spine and making sure that your abdominals are firm.

5   **Breathe out**, opening your top knee but keeping your feet connected. Your knees should form a triangle, or clam shape. You'll be able to feel the turning out from your hip joint.

6   **Breathe in** and return your lifted leg back to the other leg.

7   Repeat **10** times on this leg, then repeat on the other side.

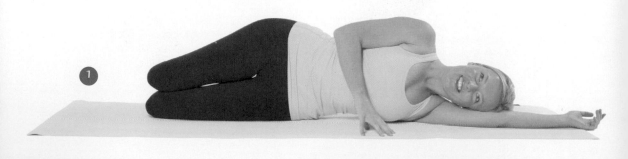

Top Tip

Keep your chest area open
throughout this move. Make sure
that your top shoulder doesn't slump
forward as you open your top leg.

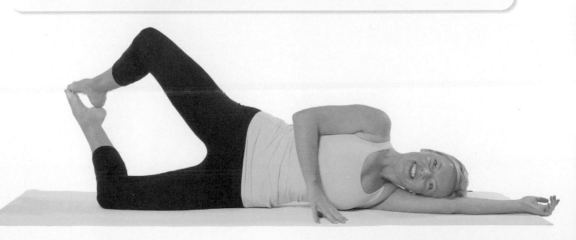

Advanced Move

If this movement feels comfortable to you, then up the ante. After you've lifted the
top leg, then use your abdominal muscle to lift your lower left leg, so that the 'clam'
shape is still formed, but both legs are off the mat. Widen the stretch if you can.

Zigzags (Sitting)

This helps to stretch and flex your hip joints. By performing this movement in the sitting position, you'll be able to maintain good stability through the spine and hips.

1   **Sit on your mat** with your knees slightly bent. Lean back to rest on your fingers. Make sure you don't overstretch your lower back.

2   **Breathe in** and slowly open your thighs to create a Y-shape in your thigh area. This movement opens up the hip joints and reinforces stability.

3   **Breathe out** and slide your legs down the mat, so that your legs are stretched fully out, reaching through your heels. Your thighs should be turned outwards, along with your feet.

Top Tip

Don't allow your knees to suddenly fall open; this will place strain on your hip joints. Instead, use slow, controlled movements.

3

4 **Stretch your feet outwards**, then inwards, creating a 'zigzag' movement with them. Your thigh muscles will also turn inwards and outwards along with your foot's movement.

5 **Bring your knees** back towards your torso, keeping your thighs and feet

turned inwards, and using your thighs to perform the move, not your back or hips.

6 **Breathe in** and turn your feet and thighs out, then slide your legs back down to the floor. Repeat the movement up to **10** times.

Toe Spread

This helps you connect your feet to your body, so that you're aware of your stance and position at all times.

1   **Sit on your mat** with a tall, neutral posture, with your pelvis and spine in neutral position and your legs straight out in front of you.

2   **Breathing normally**, flex your big toes, keeping the rest of the toes straight.

3   **Move on to** the next toe, and so on, until you've flexed each toe individually, (if possible).

4   **Reverse this**, moving from your little toe back through each toe until you reach your big toe.

5   Repeat **five** times.

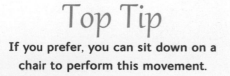

Top Tip

If you prefer, you can sit down on a chair to perform this movement.

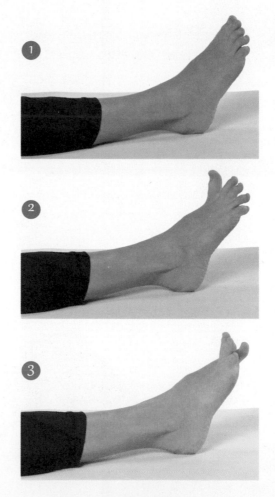

Ankle Circles

Our feet take a lot of pressure and stress, and our ankles can bear the brunt of poor posture and badly fitting shoes.

1   **Lie** in the starting position, breathing normally.

2   **Lift your left** leg towards you, placing your hands behind your knee to support the position.

3   **Your foot** should be slightly higher than your knee.

4   **Flex your foot** and begin circling it, from the ankle joint, in a clockwise direction.

5   **When you have repeated** this **five** times in one direction, repeat the movement in the opposite direction.

6   **Lower** your foot to the mat.

7   **Raise your right leg** and repeat the exercise.

The Next Level

Well done! Now that you've completed the beginner exercises, it's time to move on to more advanced exercises. These exercises take into account that you're now able to find neutral position naturally and can perform the previous movements without losing stability within the pelvis and spine.

Can Anybody Do These Movements?

If you've managed to incorporate the previous exercises into your regular exercise routine and feel comfortable doing them, it's time to move onwards and upwards. If you suffer from lower-back pain, hip discomfort or any other type of soreness, then check with your GP before advancing.

What Are These Movements For?

The next level will provide further challenges to your fitness and stability, helping to build your mobility and strength, as well as confidence in your Pilates workout. Remember that these exercises are much more difficult than the

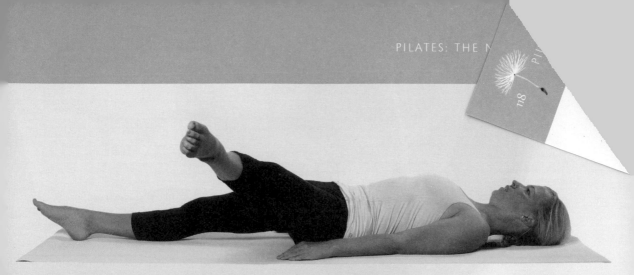

beginner's regime, so, as always, take your time with each movement. It may be an idea to attend a class that incorporates the following movements, as this can help you to pinpoint any you may find difficult or that challenge you more than others.

Let's Get Started

Try the following exercises just once each before building up to the recommended number of repetitions. In time, these movements will become much easier and you'll be able to incorporate them naturally into your Pilates routine.

As with the beginner exercises, you'll need your Pilates mat, some water and a small Pilates pillow. So let's turn the page and get moving!

The Hundred

This is quite a challenging exercise, which tests your abdominal, as well as hip and leg strength. It's ideal to release stress in your upper body.

1 **Lie on your back** with your legs bent so that your lower legs are parallel to the floor. Inhale.

2 **Exhale**. Bring your head up with your chin down and, using your abdominal muscles, curl your upper spine up off the floor to the base of your shoulder blades. Keep the shoulders sliding down and engaged in the back. Your gaze is down into the scoop of your abs.

3 **Remain here and inhale**. At the same time, deepen the pull of the abs and extend your arms and legs, so that your legs reach towards where the wall and ceiling meet in front of you. You can adjust them higher if need be, or lower for more advanced work.

2

Top Tip

If this movement is initially too difficult don't despair. To make it easier until you've had more practice, keep your head flat on the ground, but still perform the arm movements.

4 **Your legs should only be** as low as you can go without them shaking and without the lower spine pulling up off the mat. Extend your arms so that they're just a few inches off the floor, with the fingertips reaching for the far wall.

5 **Hold this position**. Take five short breaths in and five short breaths out. While doing so, move your arms in a controlled up-and-down manner – a small but dynamic pumping of the arms. Be sure to keep your shoulders and neck relaxed. It's the abdominal muscles that should be doing all the work.

3

Roll Back

This is the reverse of a roll-up (see page 124), and both are a great way to massage the spine, work the abdominals and stabilize the hips.

1 **Sit on your mat**, balanced equally on your buttocks. Your legs should be slightly apart and your feet flexed. Reach your arms out in front of you so that they're parallel to the floor and equal to your shoulder height.

2 **Your back** should be straight and your head held high. Breathe in to prepare your body.

Top Tip

Make sure that you don't hunch your shoulders over as you lower your body towards the floor. Keep your chest area open and clear.

3 **Breathe in** and slightly tuck your tummy in, creating a C-curve with your spine. Your head should be slightly bent forwards, while reaching fully through your fingertips.

4   **Breathe in to check your posture**, then breathe out and slowly begin to lower your upper body.

5   **Continue to lower** your back to the floor, keeping your arms steady and in line with your ears.

6   **Lie on the mat** with your feet pointing towards the ceiling, your arms stretched out behind you. Hold this position for the count of two, breathing in, then exhale and return to the starting position.

Roll Up

This movement looks like an advanced sit-up, but it does place a lot of pressure on your abdominal muscles and lower back. It is very important to take this exercise slowly and only reach as far as you physically can.

1 **Lie on your back** on your mat, with your feet pointing towards the ceiling, your arms stretched out behind you.

2 **Your pelvis** should be in neutral, abdominal muscles fully engaged. Breathe in to prepare and concentrate on the coming movement.

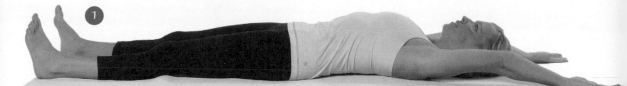

3 **Slowly lift your head** towards your chest, lifting your arms at the same time. As you bring your body up from the mat, keep your arms in line with your ears.

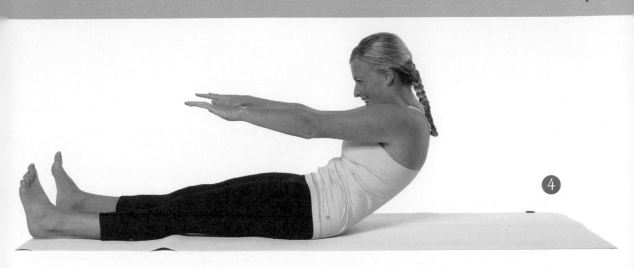

4   **Breathe out** and continue your trajectory forwards, making sure that your thighs aren't lifting off the floor.

5   **As you reach** sitting position, slowly bend forwards, so that your spine resembles a C-curve, as you tuck your stomach slightly inwards.

6   **Reach as far forwards** as you can, so that your fingertips are over, or close to, your toes. Hold this position for a couple of breaths, then slowly return to the starting position.

Top Tip

If this is too difficult for you, then just raise your head and arms and reach forwards with your arms, so that they're diagonal to your body. As you become stronger and more flexible, work your way up to the full movement.

Spine Stretch

This movement extends the spine and back, as well as the backs of the thighs.

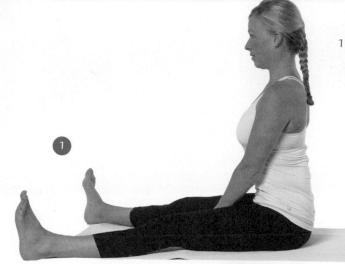

1   **Sit with your legs straight** and spread a little wider than the width of your hips. You can bend your legs if you can't sit up straight with your legs straight. Inhale and sit up as tall as you can from the base of your spine.

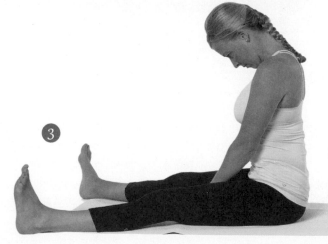

2   **Flex your feet** and reach through your heels to engage your leg muscles. Your arms should be shoulder-width apart and placed in front of you, with your palms facing down.

3   **Exhale** and drop your chin to your chest, maintaining your straight spine.

4   **Breathe in**, stretching forwards,
imagining that you're lifting your
belly up over a barrel.

Top Tip

**Keep your pelvis still – check that
you remain balanced on your sitting
bones and you don't sway from side
to side or move forwards.**

5   **Continue this stretch** as your reach
further forwards between your legs.
Don't worry if you can't touch the
ground without bending or lifting your

legs, just reach as far as you can while
keeping your legs flat on the mat.

6   **Breathe out** and return to the starting
position, sitting tall with your arms
extended out in front of you.

7   Repeat **five** times.

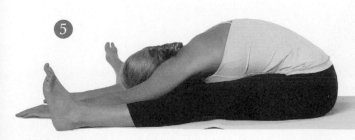

Roll Over

A fantastic all-over body stretch and massage that also helps to develop your body strength.

1   **Lie on your back** with your arms by your sides, palms facing downwards. Keep your neck long with lots of space between your shoulders and ears, and keep your chest open.

2   **With your legs together**, extend them straight up towards the ceiling at a 90-degree angle from the hips. Breathe out and lower your legs slightly. This will help to prepare your body for the rolling action.

Top Tip

Be careful not to use your back or legs to lift your legs up. The movement should come from your abdominal muscles. If this is too difficult, bring your knees to a bent position before straightening them out.

2

3   **Breathe in** and strengthen your
abdominals as you return your legs
to upright. Make sure that this
effort is coming from your abs,
not by pressing your arms or
shoulders into the ground.

3

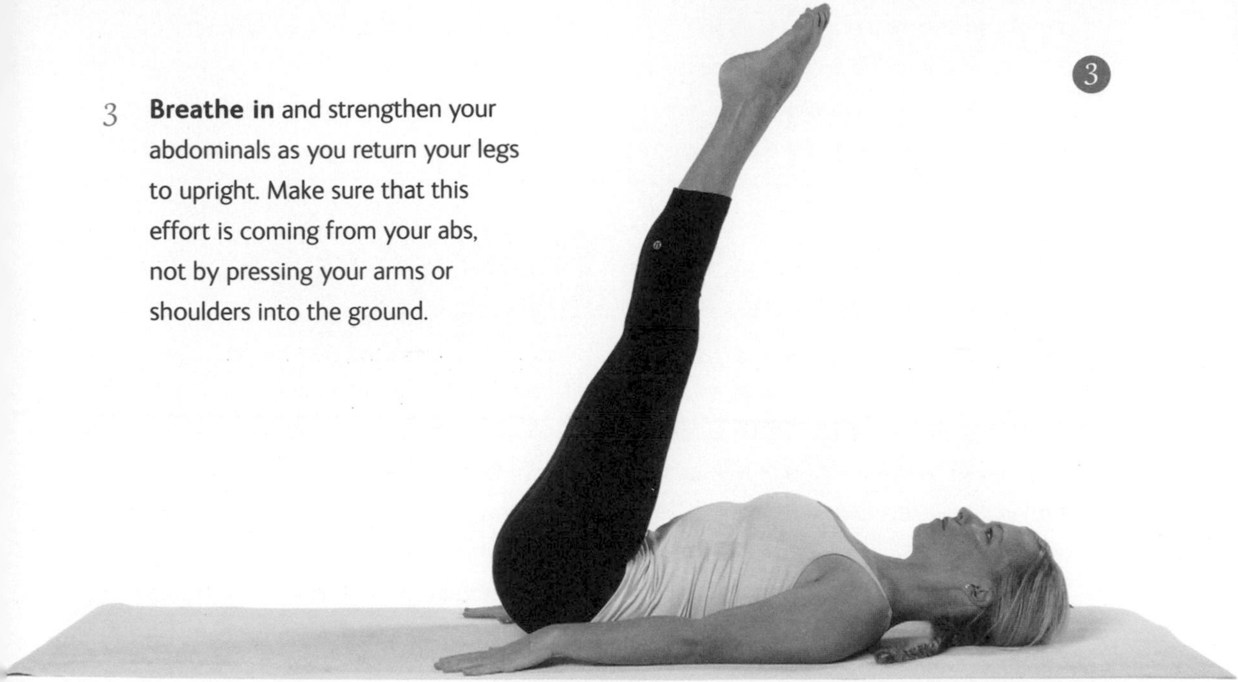

4   **Breathe out** and draw your hips
and legs over, until your legs are
parallel to your chest. You should
feel a release in your lower back
as you do so.

4

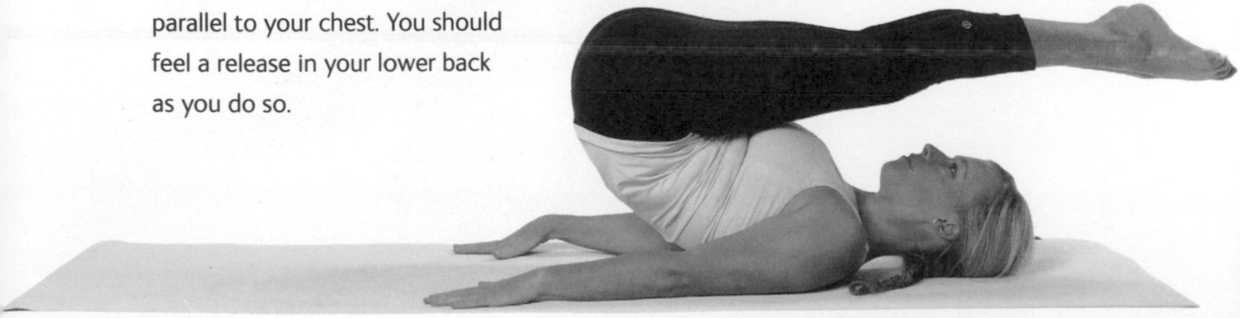

5 **Apply pressure** along the backs of your arms and palms to help continue moving your legs over your head. Your legs should be parallel to the ground and feet flexed.

6 **Breathe in** and return your legs back towards the ceiling and lower your back towards the mat.

7 **Continue lowering** your legs towards the mat, keeping your abdominal muscles firm and your shoulders lowered.

8 **Breathe out** and return your legs back over your head, using your arms if necessary to propel the movement.

9 **Breathe in** and, as your feet near the ground, point your toes towards the back of the mat. If possible, take your feet to the ground, but don't worry if this isn't possible yet.

10 **Breathe out** and slowly return to the starting position.

11 Repeat **three** times.

12 **To return your legs** to the ground, breathe in and slowly lower your legs to the mat. If this hurts your lower back too much, bend your knees and place your feet on the mat to finish.

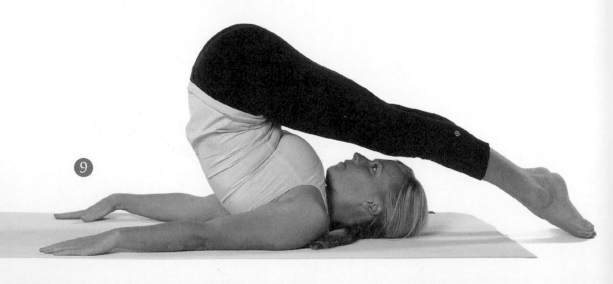

Leg Circles

This teaches your leg to move independently of your hip joint, while keeping your pelvis and spine stable. It also releases any tension in your lower back.

1   **Lie in the starting position** with your pelvis and spine in neutral.

2   **Breathe in to prepare**. As you breathe out, engage your centre and float one knee in towards your chest. Breathing with the movement, straighten your leg towards the ceiling, turning the leg out slightly from the hip and keeping your knee soft.

3   **Continue to stretch** your left leg back towards your head, then slowly circle in towards the starting position, slightly

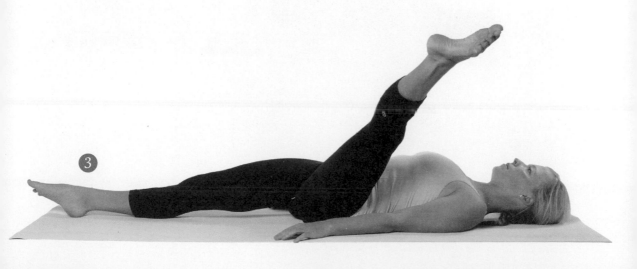

lowering your leg as you do so. If you imagine drawing a circle on the ceiling with your toes this will help you maintain the stretch. Slowly lower your leg until it's either almost touching the mat, or touching the mat, depending on your strength. Repeat.

4 **Repeat** up to **eight** times, then reverse the circles.

5 **Bend and float** your leg back to the starting position and repeat with your other leg.

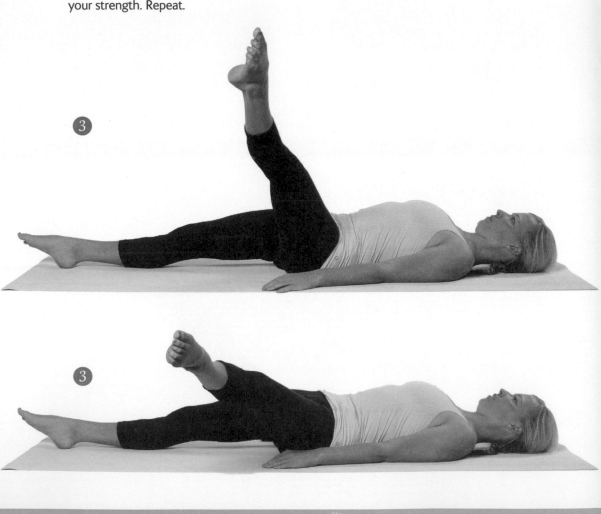

Rolling Like A Ball

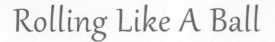

This is a lovely movement to do, especially if you want a back and spinal massage. It's important to keep your back curved constantly throughout the movement.

1   **Sit on your mat** and clasp your hands over your shins, just above the ankles. Your toes should be pointed.

2   **Drop your shoulders**, breathe in and feel your back widen. Tuck your abdominals in, while making a curve with your spine. Don't drop your head to your chest; it should stay in position so that your eyes are focusing on your knees.

3   **Lift your feet** off the mat and balance on, or just behind, your sitting bones.

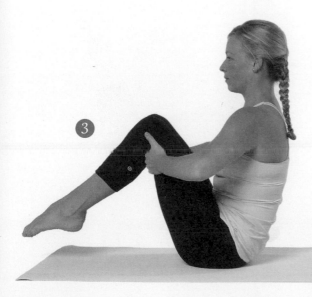

Top Tip

If this hurts your spine, place a blanket on the mat, or place two mats on top of each other for further support.

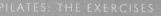

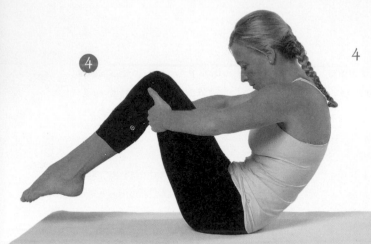

4

4 **Breathe in** and pull your lower abdominals in, as you roll on to your back. Roll on to your shoulders, not your neck, as you don't want to damage your neck bones.

5 **Pause very slightly here**, then use your outward breath and your abdominals to rock your body back to the sitting position.

6 Repeat the process **five** times.

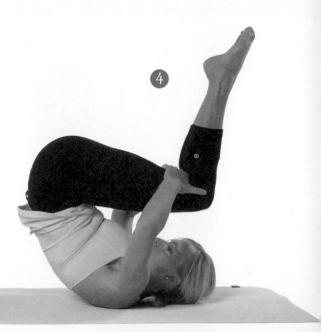

4

Open Leg Rocker

This movement can be quite difficult to do, as it challenges your stability. Perform the movement slowly, so that you don't fall to one side.

1   **Sit up tall on your mat**, balanced evenly on your sitting bones with your knees bent so that you can grasp your ankles. Lean back slightly, so that you're balanced between your sitting bones and tail bone. Keep your abdominals activated as you lift and extend one leg, then the other, to a little less than shoulder-width apart.

2   **As you breathe in**, use a deepening scoop of the abdominals and the fullness of your inhalation to propel your roll back on to your back. Bring your right leg back with you as you roll downwards, keeping your left leg stretched out. Stay in your C-curve as you roll, leaving your head and neck off the mat.

3   **Breathe out** and pause briefly here. Stay in this position and, using your abdominal muscles, bring yourself back to the upright position.

4   Repeat up to **five** times, then switch legs.

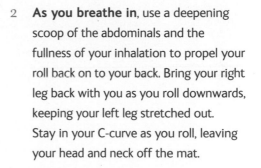

2

Spine Twist

This is a great stretch for the muscles in your back, as well as helping to keep your pelvis stable.

1   **Sit on your mat** with your back tall, balanced evenly on your sitting bones. Pull your abdominals in so that your upper body is well supported.

2   **Flex your feet** and stretch out through your heels.

3   **Extend your arms** directly out to the sides, keeping them even with your shoulders, so that there is one long line from fingertip to fingertip.

4   **Think of your spine** as being very long, with energy moving down into the floor through the tailbone and up to the sky through the top of your head. Even

with all that height, you still want to keep your shoulders relaxed and your ribcage down.

5   **If your hamstrings** are tight and it is hard for you to sit upright, place a small pillow or folded towel under your hips.

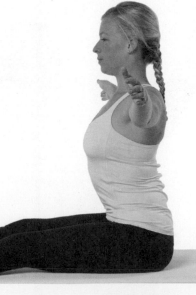

6   **Think of an imaginary line** running straight up through the middle of your body. Breathe out twice, in short gusts, feeling yourself get taller as you turn your torso and head on that central axis.

7   **The movement** is executed in two parts, where you exhale to twist halfway, then exhale again to turn as far as you can.

8   **The twist is from the waist**, not from the shoulders. The upper body, including the head, moves as one piece. The pelvis stays stable and does not twist at all. You can check this by making sure that your feet stay even with each other.

9   **Use your inhalation** to return to the centre. As you return, continue to extend energy out through your fingertips, through your heels and out of the top of your head. Control the motion and make sure that your pelvis does not move.

10   **On the exhalation**, take the twist to the other side.

11   **Repeat** the exercise **five** times on each side.

Saw

This movement is a great way to improve your Pilates breathing, while stretching your spine and the backs of the legs.

1   **Sit on your mat** with your pelvis and spine in neutral. Focus on your posture, checking that you're sitting up strong and tall.

2   **Extend your legs out** in front of you, almost shoulder-width apart.

3   **Stretch your arms** out to your sides, so that they're even with your shoulders.

4   **Breathe in**, drawing your spine up taller. Firm up your abs and turn your torso to the left, allowing your head to follow the movement.

4

5   **Breathe out** and slowly drop your chin towards your chest. Bend over your left leg, slightly twisting your spine as you do so. Reach your right arm across your left leg as if you are trying to 'saw' off your little toe.

6   **With your left arm**, reach backwards, pressing your hand away in the opposite direction to your right arm. You should feel a stretch in your spine.

7   **Pulse forwards three times**, slightly increasing the stretch and twist with each pulse. **Breathe out heavily** with each pulse, feeling all the air leave your lungs.

8   **Breathe in** and bring yourself upright, with your spine still twisted, left and right arm stretched out in front of and behind you respectively.

9   **Switch arms** over and repeat on the opposite side.

10 Repeat **five** times on each side.

Top Tip

Having trouble reaching your toes? Don't worry, just take it slowly, and gradually, with each out breath, stretch a little further forwards. Good breathing helps your muscles to relax and your stretches go further.

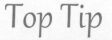

6

Back Extension

Also known as 'cobra', this yoga-inspired move helps to stretch your back, tone your abs and open your hip area.

1 **Lie on your front** on your mat, with your hips even and your spine in neutral. Rest your head on the mat, with your arms bent to either side of your head.

2 **Breathe out** and engage your abdominal muscles in preparation to move.

3 **Breathe in** and, using your arms to aid the movement, slowly bring your upper body upwards, beginning with your forehead, then breastbone, ribcage and abs. Stretch through your arms and feel the front of your body stretch.

4 **Breathe out** and slowly reverse the lift, lowering your body, first with the abs, then ribcage, breastbone, then forehead.

5 **Repeat** up to **eight** to **10** times.

Top Tip

When you return to the starting position, rest here and press your body into the floor to help release any pressure in your spine before repeating the move.

Single Leg Kick

This looks like an easy move, but it works your abdominals and upper thigh muscles. Take it slowly, as it's easy to move too quickly and cause damage to your lower back.

1 **Lie on your stomach** with both legs together, extended behind you. Activate your inner thighs and hamstrings to keep your legs from splaying out.

2 **Lift your upper body** so that you are supported on your forearms. Keep your shoulders and shoulder blades down and your chest open. Your elbows should be directly under your shoulders.

3 **Clasp your hands together** on the floor in front of you or make a fist. Your head should be in neutral, with your gaze focused on the mat. Feel the long stretch in your spine.

4 **Push your tailbone** down towards the floor as you lift your abs slightly up and away from the mat.

5 **Exhale and bend** your left leg towards your bottom until it's at a 90-degree angle to the floor. Then, pulse it twice towards your bottom with the foot

slightly pointed. Use two sharp exhales
to pulse the leg. Don't kick too hard
or you may cause pain in your
hamstrings or your lower back.

6　**Breathe in** and switch legs, so that
your left leg is extended on the mat
and your right leg is at a 90-degree
angle. Again, perform two pulses
with the right leg.

7　**Repeat** up to **five** times on each leg.

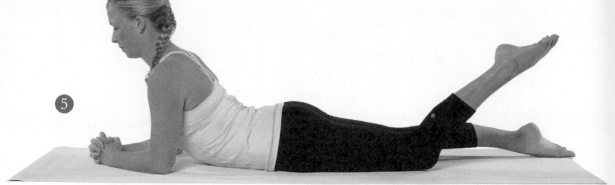

Double Leg Kick

If you suffer from lower-back pain, particularly at the end of a long day, try to do this move before you go to bed. It'll strengthen the back muscles, while releasing any tension in the area.

1   **Lie face down** on the mat in neutral position. Keep your legs together.

2   **Place your arms** behind your back, hands clasped.

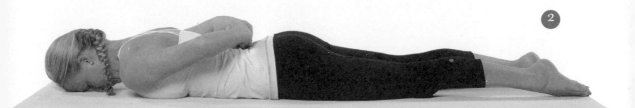

3   **Breathe in**, pulling your abdominals in while anchoring your pubic bone to the mat to help prevent any movement.

This will also help to create a nice length in your spine.

4 **Breathe out**; as you do so, kick both your legs, with your toes pointed, towards your bottom. Make sure that your hips stay stable, otherwise you'll put too much pressure on your lower back.

5 **Return your legs** to the mat. Breathe in and lift your upper body high off the mat, stretching out through the abs and chest, feeling your body lengthen. Your arms will still be behind your back – feel the lovely stretch in your chest.

6 **Breathe out** and return to the starting position.

7 Repeat **three** to **five** times.

Plank

This movement is ideal for strengthening your abdominal muscles and opening the shoulder and chest area. Build up the length of time you hold this pose to help build up your core.

1 **Kneel on the mat** with your hands on the floor in front of you, fingers pointing straight ahead. Your knees should be slightly apart, toes pointing away from your body.

2 **Breathe out** and engage your abdominals and lengthen your spine, extending the stretch through the top of your head and down through your tailbone. Lean forwards slightly to put your weight on your hands. Align your shoulders directly over your wrists.

3 **Breathe in** and, keeping your body steady, stretch your left leg behind you,

resting your feet on your toes, so that you feel a stretch through your feet all the way up through your left leg.

4 **Bring your right leg** beside your left leg, repeating the same movements.

5 **Breathe out** and bring your left leg back to the starting position. Take a couple of breaths here, then repeat the above movement on the opposite leg.

6 Repeat up to **five** times.

Side Plank

An extension of the plank move, this opens up your chest, shoulders and hips, while challenging your abdominal stability.

1 **Sit sideways** with your legs folded to the left-hand side. Put your top foot on the floor in front of the other, heel to toe. Your right arm should be out to your side, slightly wider than your shoulder.

2 **Breathe in** to prepare and lengthen your spine.

3 **As you breathe out**, activate your abdominals and press yourself into position, lifting up through your hips. Your body should be in a long line from the top of your head to your toes.

4 **Lift your left arm** up towards the ceiling, then above and over your head. Keep your fingertips stretched and feel the complete stretch all the way through your arm.

5 **Hold this position** for a couple of relaxed breaths, then return your arm to your side before lowering your hips to the ground.

6 Repeat **five** times on your left side before repeating on your right side.

Side Plank Leg Lift

Take the plank exercise even further with this challenging movement, which tests your pelvic stability while strengthening your abdominals and arms. Take your time with this movement – the more slowly you move, the more easily you'll be able to keep your balance.

1 **Begin in the side-plank starting position**, feet on top of each other, right arm out to the side, supporting your body.

2 **Breathe out** and focus on strengthening your body, stabilizing your pelvis and spine, while elongating your neck and lower back. You should feel lovely and elongated.

3 **Breathe in** and lift up through your hips, so that your body is in a line. Keep your head focused forwards. If you need help balancing, focus on an area just in front of you.

4 **Lift your left leg**, then your left arm, so that your body has

created a star shape. Do this slowly so that you don't overbalance.

5 **Hold this pose** for the count of five breaths, taking it slowly and evenly.

6 **Return** to the starting position. Repeat up to **10** times.

7 **Repeat** the movement on the other side.

4

Side Plank Leg Pull Back

Build up your thigh strength while opening up your lower-back area.

1 **Lie on your right side** with your lower arm stretched out underneath your ear. Your knees should be bent at a 90-degree angle, feet stacked on top of one another.

2 **In this position**, find your neutral spine and pelvis. Make sure your shoulders haven't slumped.

3 **Breathe in to prepare** and lengthen through the spine. Stretch your right leg down towards the end of the mat, while lifting your upper body up by using your right arm as support. Feel the lengthening in your spine and the opening of the area between your lower back and your hips. Flex your feet and feel your muscles in your thigh activate.

4 **Breathe out** as you kick the left leg directly backwards. As soon as you feel your spine move, stop and hold your leg in that position. This isn't a swinging movement, it's a controlled move, so don't swing from your bottom.

5 **Breathe in** and return to the starting position without resting your foot on the floor.

6 **Repeat six times** on the right leg before repeating the exercise on the left leg.

Side Kick Series: Front And Back

This helps to maintain stability, while strengthening your thigh muscles. Use a pillow between your head and shoulder if you need extra support.

1   **Lie on your right side** and line up your ears, shoulders, hips, knees and ankles. Your shoulders should be stacked (aligned with each other), as should your hips.

2   **Lightly support your head** with your hand, making sure to lift your ribs away from the mat so that your back and

neck stay in alignment. Modify this position by reaching your bottom arm straight out along the mat above your head and resting your head on it.

3   **The front hand rests firmly**, palm down, on the mat in front of your chest. Use this hand for balance, but don't

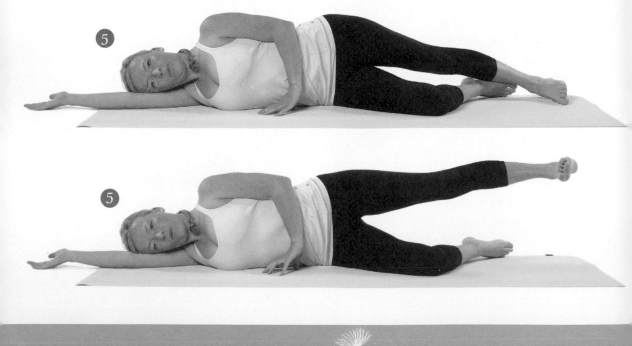

depend on it; depend on the strength of your abs.

4 **Move your legs** slightly in front of your hips. This will help stabilize your torso and protect your lower back.

5 **Rotate your legs** outwards slightly from the hips. Lift your top leg a few inches. Flex your foot and send energy out through the heel.

6 **With your foot flexed**, swing the top leg to the front. At the full length of your kick, do a small pulse kick.

7 **Keeping length in your leg** and through your whole body, point your toe and sweep your top leg to the back. Pause, but do not do a pulse kick. Only reach as far back as you can go without crunching the lower back or moving the pelvis. Again, a big part of the challenge of this exercise is to use the core muscles to keep the entire torso stable.

8 **Flex your foot** and kick to the front.

9 Repeat this exercise **five** to **10** times.

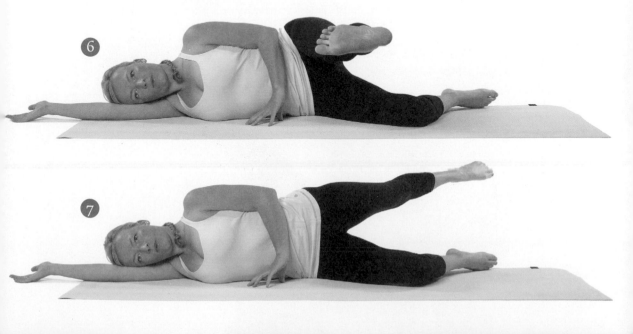

Side Kick Series: Up And Down

Open up your hip joints while building up abdominal strength. Don't take your leg too high; keep it within your comfort zone and build up your stability.

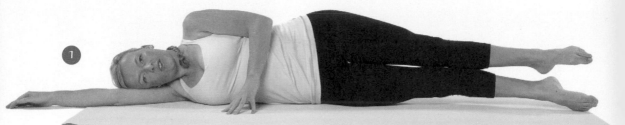

1. **Lie on your side** so that your ears, shoulders, hips, knees and ankles are all in line. Lie your head on your arm, making sure to lift the ribs away from the mat so that the back and neck stay in alignment. Rest your other hand firmly on the mat in front of your chest to help you stabilize. Make sure that your abdominal muscles are pulled in and up.

2. **Lengthening more** through the top leg, let it get so long that it moves slowly up

towards the ceiling. Make sure that the pelvis does not tilt back to let the leg go up. Keep the hipbones stacked (aligned with each other). When your leg has reached as far as it can go, flex your foot to engage your inner thigh muscles.

3 **Keep the foot flexed as your return** your leg down. Pull your abdominals up, in opposition to the lengthening of the leg, as you control the descent of the leg back to the starting position.

4 Repeat **eight** times on this leg before doing the same on the other.

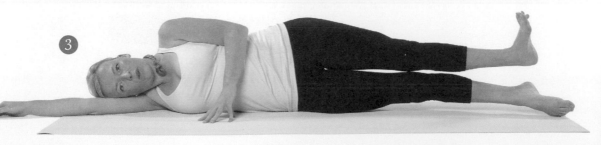

Side Kick Series: Small Circles

Open up your chest and hip area, while strengthening your inner and outer thigh muscles.

1 **Lie on your side** and line yourself up on the back of the mat with your knees bent. Your underneath arm should be supporting the side of your head and your uppermost hand should be planted firmly on the mat in front of your belly.

2 **Breathe in** and feel the stretch in your left leg as you lengthen it, keeping your toes pointed. Begin to circle your left leg in an anti-clockwise direction.

3 **Return your leg** to the starting position.

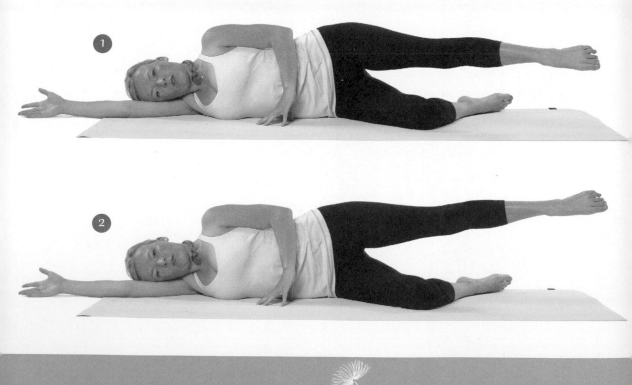

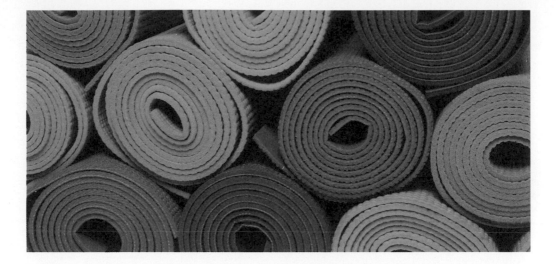

Top Tip

Keep the size of the circle about that of a watermelon. You should be able to feel the muscles in your inner and outer thighs working.

4   **Breathe out** and repeat steps 2 and 3. Try to pace yourself to one breath for each rotation.

5   **Repeat up to five times** in an anti-clockwise direction before switching to a clockwise direction.

6   **Switch sides** to perform the same movement on your right leg.

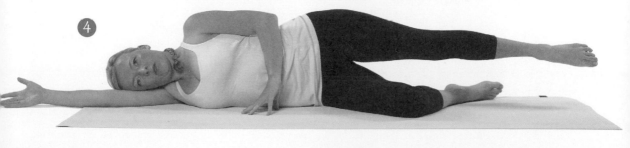

Stingray

Continue strengthening your inner thighs with this movement, which is also a lovely way to open your hips and work on stabilizing your spine and pelvis.

1 **Lie on your front** on your mat, allowing your body to rest in neutral.

2 **Breathe in** and lift your head slightly so that your shoulders are raised and less of your head is resting on the mat..

3 **Breathe in**, activating your core and, as you breathe out and lift your upper body, lengthen your legs and lift both legs slightly off the mat. Make sure that you don't experience any pain in your lower back. If you do, stop immediately.

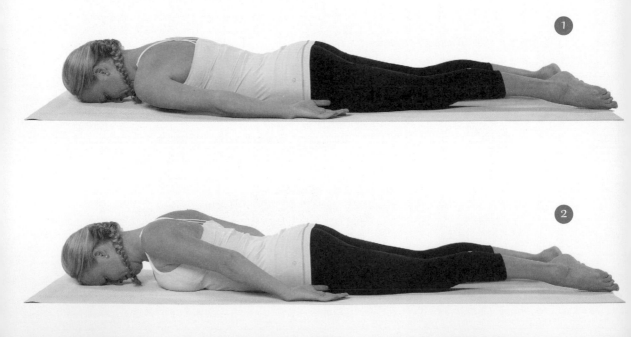

4   **Breathe out** and open your legs
    slightly, so that your thighs and feet are
    around 20 centimetres apart. Breathe
    out and, as you breathe in, beat your
    legs lightly on to the mat, taking it in
    turns, first the right leg, then the left.

5   **Breathe** evenly and beat each leg
    ten times.

Top Tip

**When you separate your
legs, turn your feet slightly
outwards, otherwise
you'll feel a strain in your
lower back.**

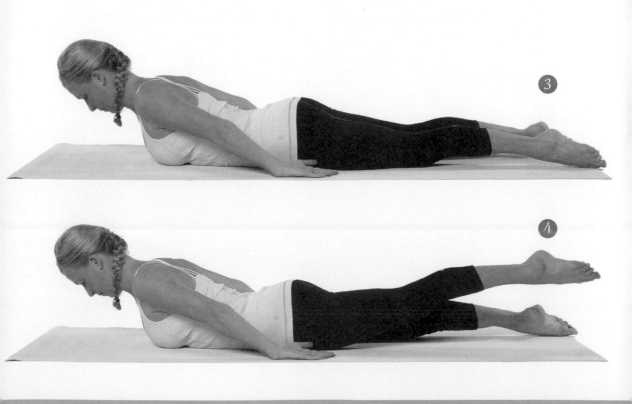

Torpedo

This helps you to lengthen the muscles in your body, while strengthening the hips. You may initially experience cramping in your hips, but as you build up your stability this should occur less.

1 **Lie in a straight line** on your side with your toes softly pointed, ensuring that your legs are not behind you. Extend your underneath arm under your head in line with your torso, and bend your top arm in front to support you.

2 **Breathe in to widen the ribcage.** Breathe out and activate your pelvic floor. Lift your top leg as high as you can without tipping your pelvis. Breathe in and bring the leg underneath up to meet your top one.

3 **Breathe out** and, squeezing both legs together, slowly lower both legs to the floor, resisting slightly with your underneath leg as you go. Repeat up to 10 times on each side, keeping your waist lengthened.

Top Tip

Use your stomach muscles, not your arm, to lift your legs. Only lift as high as you can, otherwise your upper body will become tensed and engaged.

Swimming

Strengthen your hip area with this version of the swimming exercise.

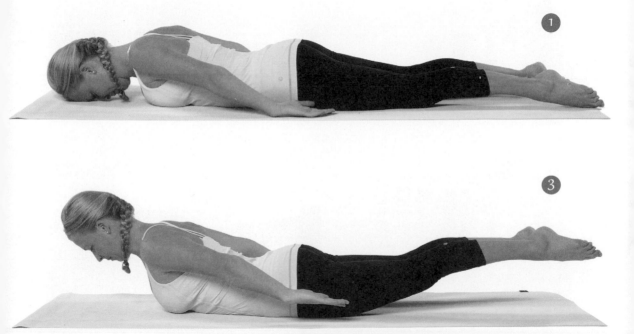

1. **Lie on your stomach**, legs straight and together.

2. **With shoulder blades settled** in your back and shoulders away from your ears, stretch your arms down your sides.

3. **Pull your abs in** so that you lift your navel away from the mat. Lift your head.

4 **Reaching from the centre**, slowly reach your arms out and towards the end of the mat, in a backwards breaststroke move. Your legs and spine should be stretched in opposite directions so that they naturally come

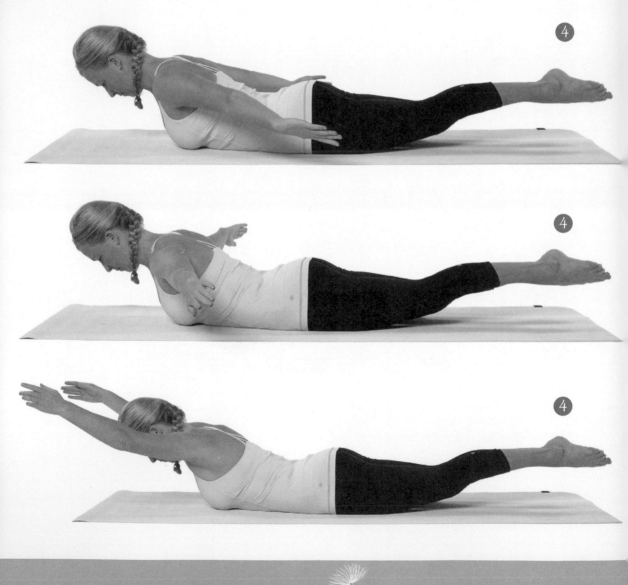

up off the floor. Keep your face and gaze directed down towards the mat.

5   **Bring your arms** back down to your side, and repeat the movement for **two** to **three** cycles.

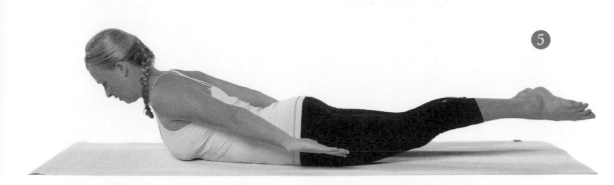

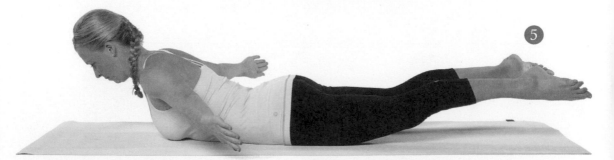

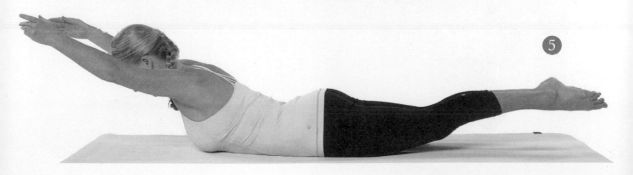

Mermaid

This opens up the spine and helps to tone and shape your waist. This is also a relaxing way to sit and stretch your hips.

1   **Sit with your left leg crossed** in front of you, the other knee bent in front of your chest, foot on the floor. Your hands should rest on your bent knee. Make sure that your spine is straight, pushing your shoulders towards the ground to elongate your neck. Fix your gaze straight ahead of you.

2   **With your left leg still** in the cross-legged position, straighten your right leg in front of you with your foot flexed and your toes pointing to the sky.

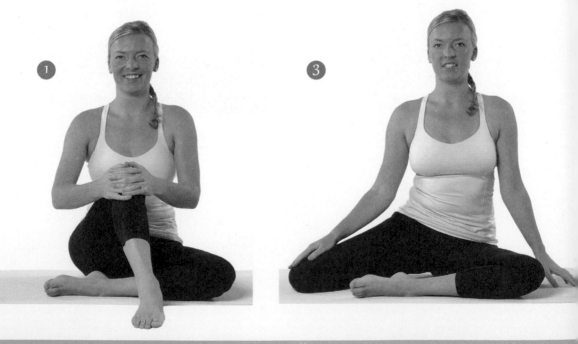

3   **Bend your right leg** and gently swing your foot behind your right buttock. The bottom of your foot should be facing up with your toes pointing behind you. Your left foot should be gently pressing against your right inner thigh.

4   **Straighten your arms** to your sides, allowing your fingertips to touch the mat either side of your body.

5   **Bend your body towards the left**, lowering your left elbow to the mat as you do so. Your gaze should be focused on your left hand, your body slightly reaching over your left hip towards your left elbow.

6   **As you inhale**, raise your right arm, gently stretching it, then curve it over your head. Make sure to keep your hips pointing straight ahead of you and planted on the ground.

7   **Slightly tilt your torso** from the waist up in the same direction as your right arm.

8   **Hold the stretch for a few seconds** and then exhale and return the right arm to your side with your palm planted on the mat.

9   **Repeat five times** on the left side and then switch to the right side.

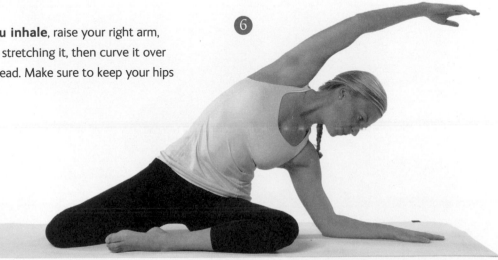

The Ultimate Level

As you become more practised and confident with the previous Pilates movements, you can move on to more challenging ones. These are not easy and it's doubtful that you'll be able to complete many on your first attempt. But persevere! It's well worth sticking to, as the advanced exercises will round off your entire Pilates experience.

A Natural Evolution

The following exercises are based on the original teachings of Joseph Pilates, but have evolved over the years. They will challenge your core and stability and can take years to perfect. You will have already noticed how much your body has changed through your regular Pilates workout. With the ultimate level, your body will become honed a little more, and your core and stability a little stronger.

Don't Give Up

If you feel that you are ready for the ultimate Pilates level, it may be time to revisit a studio or Pilates instructor. They can help assess whether

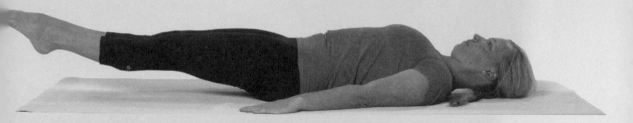

you're ready to progress, and also to double-check that you're not making any mistakes that could lead to short- or long-term injury. Your instructor can also give you further advice on the exercises in the next chapter to help you in your home workout.

About The Exercises

The ultimate Pilates level is a highly powered and revitalizing workout designed for those who are entirely comfortable with the previous movements. You should now be able to perform the previous chapter's exercises without referring to the book for assistance.

Remember, there is no rush. If you don't feel ready to move up to this level, continue to practise the movements covered up to now before moving on.

Corkscrew

Get yourself in a twist with this great spinal stretch.

1 **Lie on your back** with your shoulders away from your ears and arms along your sides, palms down. Before you begin the exercise, take a few deep breaths, allowing your belly to deepen down towards your spine and your spine to lengthen out along the mat. Your lower back will be on the mat. This is not a neutral spine exercise.

2 **Extend your legs** up to the ceiling. Keep them together, hugging the midline of the body.

3 **Breathe in**. Keeping your belly scooped in, use abdominal control to take your legs to the right side. Keep your legs together, but do not squeeze them too hard.

4 **Make this a small move** at first, keeping the hips on the mat. As you get stronger, let just the hips tip slightly to the right with the move as shown. (Eventually this exercise takes the hips all the way off the mat.)

2

5   **Your upper body** will remain calm
    and stable. Lightly press the backs of
    your arms on the mat.

6   **Circle your legs down** behind your
    head, but don't take your legs so low
    that your upper back comes off the mat.

7   **As your legs begin** to move
    to the left side of your arc,
    use your exhale to take

them around and up. You should feel a
strong deepening scoop of the lower
belly as you bring your legs around and
up to the starting position.

8   **Do another arc** in the other
    direction. Continue until you have
    done **three** to each side.

Swan Dive

This looks relatively easy, and is a great massage for your internal organs, but make sure to keep your hips and spine stable to avoid any pain or injury.

1   **Lie on your stomach**. Lift your abdominals away from the floor and send your tailbone down towards the floor, anchoring the pubic bone.

2   **Keep your legs straight**, but slightly apart. Slide your shoulder blades down your back as you place your hands under your shoulders, elbows in. Maintain a long spine as you press up.

3   **Press through and up** until your arms are straight or close to straight. It is more important to keep the length in the back, with the tailbone down and the abs lifting, than to push up high. Do not push up so high that you feel a pinch in your lower back.

Top Tip

This is a powerful exercise that uses the breath to help propel it. Try to do swan dive with a sense of flowing through one part to another, rather than as two separate movements.

3

4 **Release your arms**, extending them straight alongside your ears. Your body will rock forwards and, because you are keeping your long arc, your legs will come up. Your job is to keep your inner thighs and glutes engaged, your abs lifted and your shoulders integrated, firm and strong, alongside your core.

4

5 **Inhale**. Keep your lovely, long arc shape and use the length and reach of your body, along with intention, to rock back and forth with your arms extended out. Don't drop your upper body or all will be lost and you won't get going again. Find the move through your extension and core: glutes work, inner thighs work, back extensors and abs.

6 Repeat **three** to **five** times.

5

Neck Pull

While this looks like a typical sit-up, it's a much more difficult movement, as it challenges your abdominals to perform the movement, while keeping your pelvis stable.

1 **Begin by lying on the mat** on your back with your arms by your side. Release tension in your hip muscles and feel your whole back and body against the floor. Let the back of your lower ribs release towards the floor.

2 **Keep your legs** shoulder-width apart or together; find out what works best for you. Even if your legs are apart, you have to engage the inner thighs and inner hamstrings. If your legs are apart, keep your feet flexed.

3 **Breathe in** and leave your shoulders down as you lengthen along your spine and out the top of your head as you curl your head and shoulders off the mat. Let your chest be wide, but make sure you haven't tensed up.

4 **Breathe out** and pull your abs in deeply to continue your roll up. Don't pull with your hands; all the movement should be instigated by your core.

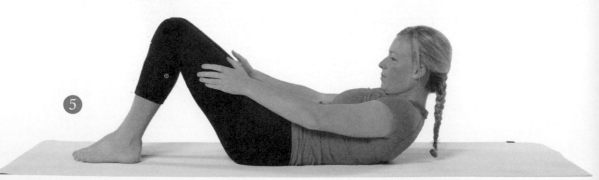

5 **If you have trouble getting up**, try a few roll ups with bent knees, feet on the floor and hands behind the thighs.

6 **Continue to exhale** to take your curved spine and lifted abs all the way over your legs. Make sure your chest has stayed open and your elbows are back in line with your ears.

7 **Breathe in** and bring your pelvis back to upright. Begin stacking your spine from the bottom up until you are sitting straight up on your sitting bones with your head relaxed. Your shoulders should have stayed down away from your ears the whole time.

8 **Exhale** and roll your spine down on to the floor.

9 **Continue to exhale** until you are all the way back to the starting position.

10 **Inhale** and repeat the exercise **three** more times.

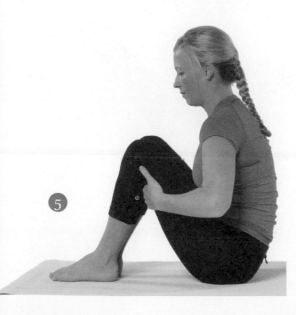

Top Tip

Take it one step further. From step 6, continue to inhale and tip back with a flat back, increasing the angle between your thighs and torso beyond 90 degrees. Don't go too far. Control the move and be sure your legs don't fly up. The point is to lengthen your spine in both directions. Connect to the floor and use that to get an amazing lift through your back and body to take you up and back. Don't just lean the upper body back so that your ribs pop open. Keep the connection down the back of the legs and through the heels.

Bicycle

It may take you some time to balance and complete this movement. While this helps to promote stability in the pelvis, torso and spine, it's also a wonderful stretch in your lower back.

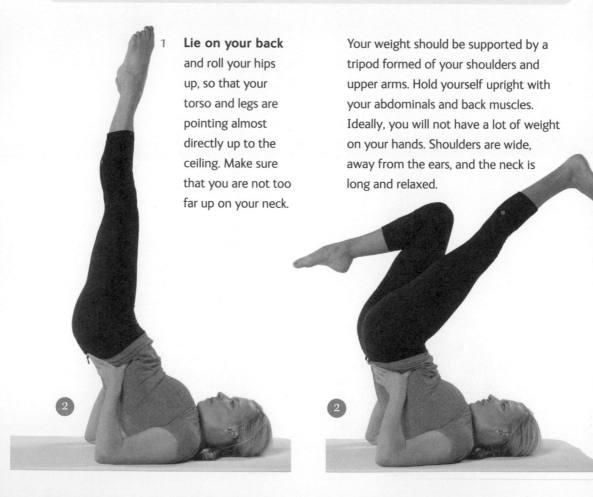

1 **Lie on your back** and roll your hips up, so that your torso and legs are pointing almost directly up to the ceiling. Make sure that you are not too far up on your neck.

Your weight should be supported by a tripod formed of your shoulders and upper arms. Hold yourself upright with your abdominals and back muscles. Ideally, you will not have a lot of weight on your hands. Shoulders are wide, away from the ears, and the neck is long and relaxed.

2   **Bend the right knee** and extend the left leg towards the wall behind you, bringing it straight over your head, until almost parallel with the floor.

3   **As each leg moves** to its fullest extension, the left leg bends to come back in the direction it came from as the right leg makes a long arc up and overhead. Basically, this is like pedalling in reverse. It makes the exercise harder and it makes you think a bit more too.

Top Tip

As you get more comfortable with this movement, you can take the legs even further apart so that eventually they move into a wide split before one leg folds and threads past the other one as it arcs towards the ceiling.

4   **Do up to 10 sets** of reverse pedalling, then bring the legs together and use abdominal control to roll back down.

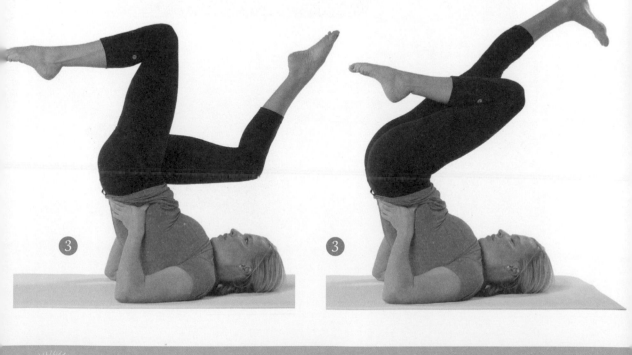

Scissors

This movement may take you some time to perfect, but it's worth it. It's an ideal stretch for your lower back, and promotes stability in your hips and spine.

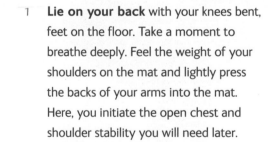

1 **Lie on your back** with your knees bent, feet on the floor. Take a moment to breathe deeply. Feel the weight of your shoulders on the mat and lightly press the backs of your arms into the mat. Here, you initiate the open chest and shoulder stability you will need later.

2 **Bring your knees** towards your chest and bring your head towards your knees, so that your shoulders are slightly off the mat.

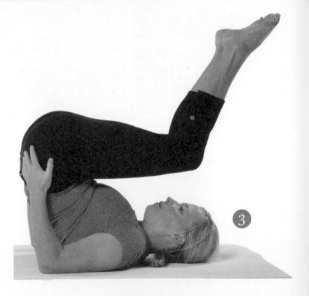

3   **Roll your hips up** off the mat so that you are in an upside-down ball position, resting on your shoulders. Cup the back of your pelvis with your hands and have your elbows directly under your hips.

4   **Extend your hips** and your legs so you are diagonal. Make sure your chest is still open and your neck is relaxed. Drop your shoulders if you need to, and get support from the backs of the upper arms.

5   **Scissor your legs open**, moving them in opposite directions. The tendency is to bring the overhead leg too far back. Just take it as far as you *comfortably* can.

6   **Scissor the legs twice** in the open position. Make sure that only the legs move. The pelvis should stay completely stable.

7   **Repeat** the scissor action **six** times.

8   **Bring your legs together** overhead and roll down slowly, in a controlled manner.

Shoulder Bridge

Stretch your lower back while strengthening your stomach muscles and thighs. This will also challenge your pelvic stability.

1 **Lie on your back** in neutral spine, with your knees bent and feet on the floor. Your legs are hip-width apart and parallel. Your arms are extended along your sides. Press the backs of your arms into the mat.

2 **Breathe in** and press down through your feet to lengthen your spine and press your hips up. Come to a bridge position on your shoulders with your knees, hips and shoulders in one line. Your abs and hamstrings should be engaged.

3 **Pause at the top** of the bridge to practise lifting one leg, then the other, off the mat.

4 **Breathe in** and fold one knee in towards your chest and then extend that leg towards the ceiling. The rest of the body stays still. Relax your shoulders and neck; the work is in the abs and hamstrings.

5 **Breathe out** and lower your leg so that your knees are side by side. As you lower your leg, go for as much length as you can. The knee of your supporting leg, the extended leg, and the tailbone are reaching for the wall in front of you as the top of your head is reaching away in an oppositional stretch.

2

6   **Inhale and flex** your foot and kick your leg up to the ceiling again. Be sure that your hips remain even and that the hip of the working leg does not try to lift up along with the kick.

7   **Exhale** and bring your working knee back to your chest and return your foot to the floor.

> ## Top Tip
> This movement should be controlled and flowing, with an easy co-ordination of movement and breath.

8   **Roll down** through your spine to return to your starting position.

9   **Repeat this exercise two** to **three** times on each side.

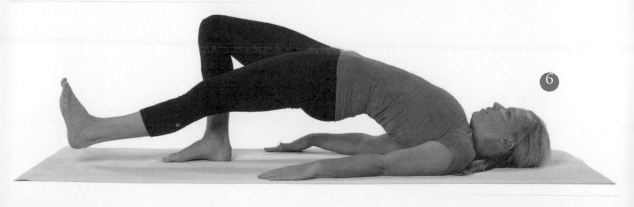

Jackknife

Another great way to stretch your lower back and strengthen your shoulders. Use your arms to support your movement if needed.

1   **Lie on your back** with your arms by your sides, palms down. Lightly press the backs of your arms into the mat and open your chest. Your ribs stay down. Imprint your spine on to the mat as you extend your legs, feet towards the ceiling.

2   **Inhale** and use a deepening scoop of your abdominal muscles and some help from the press of your arms to bring your legs over your head, parallel to the floor. Your back is nicely curved so that the weight is across your shoulders and not on your neck.

3   **Exhale and keep your chest open** and shoulders down as you sweep your legs up so that you are as close as you can get to perpendicular to the floor.

Check that you are resting on your shoulders, not your neck, getting help from the press of your shoulders and arms on the mat. Hold this position at the top of the movement.

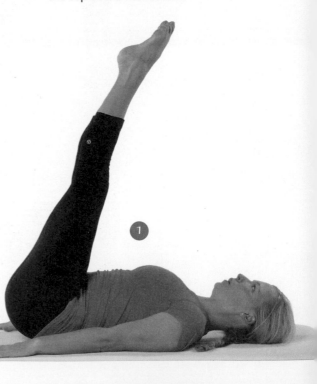

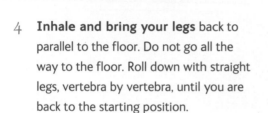

2

3

4 **Inhale and bring your legs** back to
parallel to the floor. Do not go all the
way to the floor. Roll down with straight
legs, vertebra by vertebra, until you are
back to the starting position.

5 **Repeat** the exercise **two** more times.

4

Side Kick Series: Side Passé

Keep your hips as stable as possible to help lengthen and strengthen your spine.

1 **Lie on your left side**, so that there is a straight line from your head to your toes. Place your right hand behind your head and lean on your left elbow. Toes should be pointed.

2 **Breathe in** and lift your right leg directly up, so that your foot is pointed towards your knee.

3   **Breathe out** and slide your foot down the length of the bottom leg until it is straight and hovering at hip height, then lift the leg up to the ceiling, before lowering it back down.

4   **Repeat three to five times** and then reverse the movement. Bend the knee, sliding the foot up the inside of the thigh. Extend the leg straight to the ceiling. Lengthen your leg from the hip socket and then lower it back down to meet the bottom leg.

5   Repeat **three** to **five** times.

Top Tip

If you find that you cramp in your hip when you do this movement, keep the opening of your leg smaller and lift it a little lower. You can rub the affected area to encourage more blood flow to help reduce the cramp too.

Teasers I, II and III

This is one of the hardest exercises for your abdominal muscles. The aim is to move as fluidly as possible to maintain stability.

Teaser I

1   **Lie on your back** with your arms by your sides. Extend your legs to a 45-degree angle. Breathe in to prepare.

2   **Exhale and lengthen** your spine to nod your head slightly and begin scooping your abdominal muscles in and up so that your upper body begins to roll off the mat. Simultaneously reach your arms so they are coming up to parallel with your legs. Your fingertips should reach past your toes, but keep your shoulders down.

3   **Inhale as you come to the top** and open your chest, lifting your head slightly to fully extend the length of your spine.

4   **Exhale to roll down**. Start from the low abs and use control, rolling down

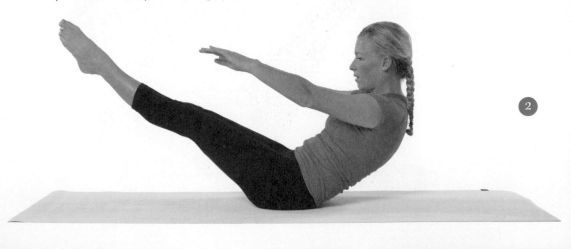

2

sequentially along the spine. Keep the legs together. Think of rolling down your midline. Repeat **three** times.

Teaser II

1   **Breathe in** and, from step 1 from Teaser I, stay strong and lift the upper body. Keeping your legs controlled, lengthen your arms above your head in line with your ears. Keep your eyes focuseds forward and chest lifted.

2   **Breathe out** and begin to roll your pelvis underneath you, keeping good control of your upper body and legs. Keep your arms lengthened above your head. Repeat up to **five** times.

Teaser III

1   **To take this movement** one step further, from step 2 of the previous movement, lower your legs a little further towards the ground, keeping your spine stable, chest lifted and abdominals strong, then draw your legs back up towards you, back into the 'V' position.

2   **Finish by rolling down**, back to the starting position.

T11₂

Kneeling Side Kicks

This move will tell you how far your stability has advanced, while helping to strengthen your hips and spine.

1 **Begin by kneeling** on your mat. Pull your abdominals in and drop your tailbone towards the floor. Your arms should be stretched out at shoulder height. Feel your arms lengthen through your fingertips.

2 **Extend your right leg** directly out to the side, with your toe on the floor. Your toes should be pointed out towards the end of the mat.

3 **Drop your left hand** to the floor, directly under your shoulder, leaving your arm straight. This will take your torso to the side. Place your right hand behind your head with your bent elbow pointing towards the ceiling. Flex your

foot and swing your right leg to the
front. At the full length of your kick, do
a small pulse kick, feeling the stretch
along the back of your leg.

4   **Keeping length** in your leg and
extension through your whole body,
point your toe and sweep your top leg
to the back. Pause, but do not do a
pulse kick.

5   **This is a smooth exhalation**. Only
reach as far back as you can go without
losing your alignment. You may find this
to be a good hip opener.

6   **Repeat the
exercise six** to **eight**
times on each side.

Top Tip

**If it's too difficult to swing your leg
forwards, then lift and stretch it
out to the side, around hip height.**

Side Twist

An intense, complicated movement, which will require a certain level of practice before it becomes simpler.

1   **Sit on your mat** on your right hip, leaning on your right hand, palm facing downwards. Fold your left leg in front of your right leg. Place your left arm on your ankle or calf of your bent left leg.

2   **Breathe in as you begin** to lift your hip, reaching with your left arm over your head, with your fingertips pointing down towards the mat.

3   **Breath out** as you turn your head and chest and twist towards the mat. Keep your left arm by your head and feel your spine stretch, curling inwards.

4   **Breathe in** as you return back, so that your spine is untwisted and your arm is stretched out over your head.

5   **Continue to breathe in** as you turn your head, chest and left arm towards the ceiling. Keep your legs touching and make sure that you haven't moved your spine or pelvis.

3

Top Tip

Check your feet. They should be placed slightly in front of each other, with your legs keeping contact at all times.

6 **Exhale and return your arm**, head and chest to the centre before bending the knees, circling the left arm down and returning to the starting position.

7 **Repeat up to five times**, then swap sides and repeat **five** times on the other side.

5

Rocking

This is a lovely rocking motion, which massages the lower back while challenging and strengthening the abdominal muscles. Keep the movement controlled so that you don't lose your balance.

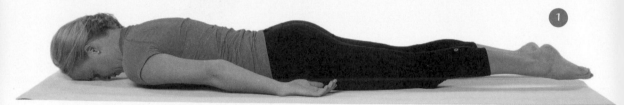

1

1   **Lie on your stomach**, nose to the floor and your arms by your sides. Take a moment to lengthen your spine and engage your abdominal muscles. Bring your mind to focus on your core.

2   **Keep your head down for now.** Bend one knee and grasp your ankle.

Bend the other knee and grasp that ankle. As much as possible, keep your legs parallel throughout the exercise, so you must engage your inner thighs.

3   **Inhale and press your ankles** into your hands as you simultaneously lift your chest and knees away from the mat. This is a long back extension with

2

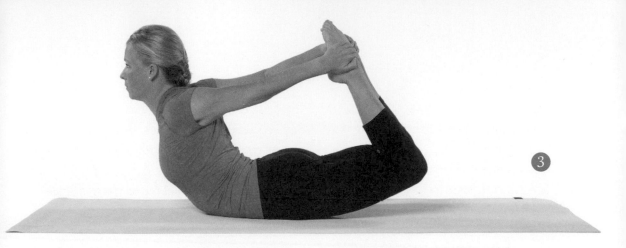

your neck extending through your shoulder girdle as your arms reach back, your chest open and face forwards.

4   **Now add the rocking part** of the exercise. Hold the beautiful crescent shape you created in step 3. Keep your legs as close to parallel as you can. Exhale to rock forward. Inhale to lift. The rocking is accomplished mostly with the breath and subtle shifts in the way you use your abdominal and back muscles – much like you do in the swan dive (*see* page 168).

5   **Once you get going**, you can exaggerate the movement to get a high lift of the legs as you rock forward, and a high, open chest as you rock back.

Stretching and Cool Down

It's very important to stretch properly. When you work your muscles, the 'elastic bands' inside the muscle bunch and can knot. If you don't give your brain notice of operating a muscle at a certain length by stretching it, you run the risk of walking around with it in an unready state and straining it. You'll also feel more graceful once your brain is in a state of preparedness and knows you're about to get physical.

After a workout, cool-down stretches help to return the muscles to their resting length. During activity you stress your muscles and they swell up, but they also contract, which gives them a bunched up, knotty appearance. If you don't elongate your muscles, they'll stay contracted and start restricting your everyday movements, risking joint strain and injury.

The Benefits Of Stretching

A study at the University of Michigan found elderly people benefited from stretching and that it could reduce the risk of injury. One of our biggest health problems, osteoarthritis, is caused by lack of movement and early degeneration of the joints. This causes premature wearing of the joints and arthritis. Stretching in your youth can help prevent osteoarthritis in later life.

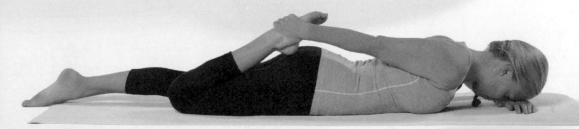

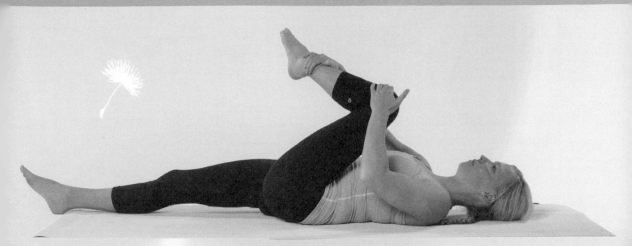

When Should You Stretch?

The jury is still out on whether you should stretch before and after a workout, but one thing is clear: warming up your muscles definitely helps your mind and body prepare for the upcoming exercises. As for cooling down... After a Pilates workout you should feel awake and invigorated. Which is perfect. However, you do still need to cool down your body and mind, particularly if you do a routine at night, otherwise you'll feel too wired to sleep. So don't rush, take your time to correctly warm up and cool down, and you'll receive the full benefits of your workout.

Hamstring Flossing

This is a great way to stretch the hamstring muscles at the backs of your thighs, while you maintain a stable and relaxed torso.

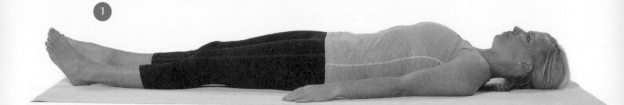

1   **Lie in the starting position**, with one or two small cushions underneath your head if needed, to enable your shoulders to relax.

2   **Lift your right leg** towards your body and hold under the knee.

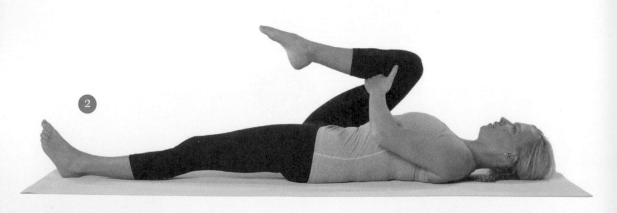

Top Tip

Stretching your hamstrings will help prevent that horrible tightness that can occur the next day after exercise. Well-stretched hamstrings will also help your legs look leaner and more toned.

③

3   **Straighten the knee.** stretching the leg further backwards. To floss, you flatten the foot, then straighten it. This puts a stretch on to the nerve and deals with the tightness around the nerve.

4   Repeat up to **10** times.

③

Quad Flossing

This takes the previous stretch a step further, helping to warm up the outer thigh areas, as well as the hips.

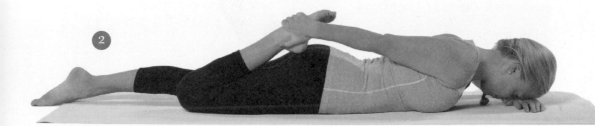

1   **Lie on your front**, legs slightly apart, head face down on your hands.

2   **Lift the right leg towards your buttocks.** Your toes should be pointed. Grasp your ankle or calf muscle.

3   **Flex your foot**, so that your toes are pointing towards the ceiling. You should feel the stretch in your lower back, bottom, thigh and shin.

4   **Return your leg** to the mat and repeat with the opposite side.

5   **Hold each stretch** for the count of eight.

Superficial Glute Stretch

A great way of stretching the muscles of your bottom, while challenging your neutral pelvis and spine.

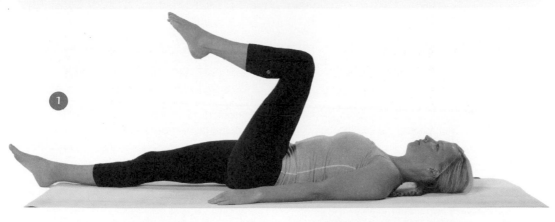

1   **Lie on your back** and bring your left leg towards your chest.

2   **Grasp your knee** (lightly) and gently pull your left leg towards your chest. Your right leg should be flat on the mat, toes pointed forwards.

3   **Hold this stretch** for the count of five, breathing normally.

4   **Return your leg** to the mat and repeat on the opposite leg.

Deep Glute Stretch

A further extension of the Superficial Glute Stretch, which also stretches the lower back.

1 **Lie in the starting position.** Breathe in to prepare and lengthen your spine. Breathe out and focus on your core and pelvis and fold your left knee into your chest. Open your knee out to the side and rest your left ankle on your right knee. Breathe in, checking your neutral spine and pelvis. Check your waist is long on both sides and your pelvis is square.

2 **Breathe out**, deepen your abdominals and fold your right leg in, bringing your left leg further towards you. Take your hands around the back of your right thigh, lacing your left arm between your legs. Gently draw in your right leg and press your left knee away from you, to deepen the stretch. Make sure your tailbone stays grounded. Breathe into the stretch for a few breaths. Return your legs to the starting position with control, and repeat on the other side.

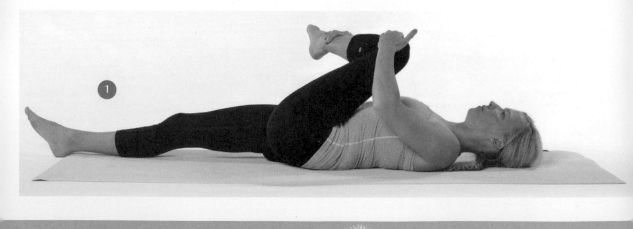

Anterior Hip Stretch

Another great way to open up the hip area and relieve any tension or soreness.

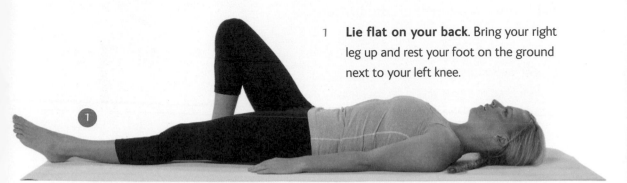

1 **Lie flat on your back**. Bring your right leg up and rest your foot on the ground next to your left knee.

2 **Bring your knee up** towards your right shoulder without rotating the lumbar spine. Place your left ankle above the right knee . If this is uncomfortable, you may place the ankle below the knee.

3 **Using your hands** clasped around your knee, gently push your right hip down into the floor until a stretch is felt in the front of your hip; contracting your right buttock will help.

4 **Hold for the count of five** and repeat on the opposite leg.

Walking Calf Stretch

Release any tension or pain in your calf muscles with this stretch. It can also be done standing against a wall if this movement is too difficult.

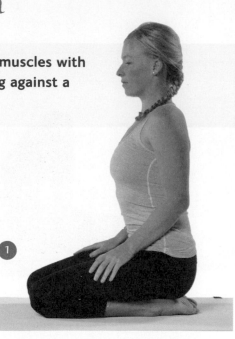

1   **Sit on your mat**, knees bent under you so that you're sitting on your feet.

2   **Lean forwards**, arms under your shoulders, feet flexed and shins off the ground.

3   **Breathe in to prepare** and breathe out, reaching forwards with your hands

and lifting your knees into a downward dog pose, so that your bottom is in the air. Your back is fully stretched with your head between your hands, looking back between your legs, and your legs are completely stretched. Your feet should be flat on the mat if possible.

3

4   **Bend your elbows slightly** and lift your right heel, as though you're going to step forwards.

5   **Place your foot back** on the mat and repeat with the left foot.

6   **Take as many steps** as you like, feeling the stretch in your legs, in particular your calves.

4

Book Openings (Side Lying)

This is a repeat of the book openings on pages 98–100, but this time you can hold the stretch for as long as you want.

1 **Lie on your left side**, knees bent, arms out in front of you, hands on top of each other. Make sure that your shoulders aren't slumped. Place a small pillow under your head if you like.

2 **Breathe in** to prepare and breathe out, lifting your right arm towards the ceiling.

3 **Continue to breathe out** and reach behind you, almost to the floor if you can.

4 **Only stretch** as far as you feel comfortable. Your head should be turned so that you're looking over your shoulder.

5 **Hold for a count** of five (or longer if you prefer) and return to the starting position.

6 **Repeat three to five times** on this side before swapping over to the right side.

Spiky Ball Massage

This helps to release tension and toxins in your thighs. You can use the spiky ball anywhere on your body to give yourself an all-over massage.

1   **Sit on your mat** with your left knee bent, right leg stretched out in front of you.

2   **Using the ball in your right hand,** gently roll it along the outside of your thigh. It may hurt slightly, but you should feel a wonderful massaging sensation. Work down towards your feet.

3   **Repeat** on the other leg.

4   **Repeat the same motion** on both arms to release any tension.

Top Tip

Use the spiky ball to massage following your morning workout. This will help to detoxify your body and stimulate your skin cells.

Checklist

Stability Exercises

- [ ] Cat Stretch
- [ ] Extended Cat Stretch
- [ ] Knee Openings
- [ ] Single Knee Openings
- [ ] Leg Slides
- [ ] Imprinting
- [ ] Arm Openings
- [ ] Overhead Arms

Basic Standing Exercises

- [ ] Floating Arms
- [ ] Tennis Ball Rising
- [ ] Standing On One Leg
- [ ] Pilates Squats
- [ ] Wrist Circles
- [ ] Dumb Waiter
- [ ] Cocktails Anyone?
- [ ] Roll Down

Basic Mat Exercises

- [ ] Shoulder Drops
- [ ] Arm Circles
- [ ] Pelvic Clocks
- [ ] Pelvic Rolls

- [ ] Bridge
- [ ] Windows
- [ ] Knee Circles
- [ ] Curl Ups
- [ ] Oblique Curl Ups
- [ ] Hip Rolls
- [ ] Table Top
- [ ] Diamond Press
- [ ] Dart
- [ ] Book Opening (Sitting)
- [ ] Book Opening (Lying)
- [ ] Arm Openings
- [ ] Single Leg Stretch
- [ ] Oblique Single Leg Stretch
- [ ] Knee Rolls
- [ ] Double Leg Stretch
- [ ] Clam
- [ ] Zigzags (Sitting)
- [ ] Toe Spread
- [ ] Ankle Circles

The Next Level

- [ ] The Hundred
- [ ] Scissors
- [ ] Roll Back

- [ ] Roll Up
- [ ] Spine Stretch
- [ ] Roll Over
- [ ] Leg Circles
- [ ] Rolling Like A Ball
- [ ] Open Leg Rocker
- [ ] Spine Twist
- [ ] Saw
- [ ] Back Extension
- [ ] Single Leg Kick
- [ ] Double Leg Kick
- [ ] Plank
- [ ] Side Plank
- [ ] Side Plank Leg Lift
- [ ] Side Plank Leg Pull Back
- [ ] Side Kick Series: Front And Back
- [ ] Side Kick Series: Up And Down
- [ ] Side Kick Series: Small Circles
- [ ] Stingray
- [ ] Torpedo
- [ ] Swimming
- [ ] Mermaid

The Ultimate Level

- [ ] Corkscrew
- [ ] Swan Dive
- [ ] Neck Pull
- [ ] Bicycle

- [ ] Shoulder Bridge
- [ ] Jackknife
- [ ] Side Kick Series: Side Passé
- [ ] Teasers I, II and III
- [ ] Kneeling Side Kicks
- [ ] Side Twist
- [ ] Rocking

Stretching And Cool Down

- [ ] Hamstring Flossing
- [ ] Quad Flossing
- [ ] Deep Glute Stretch
- [ ] Superficial Glute Stretch
- [ ] Anterior Hip Stretch
- [ ] Walking Calf Stretch
- [ ] Book Openings Side Lying
- [ ] Spiky Ball Massage

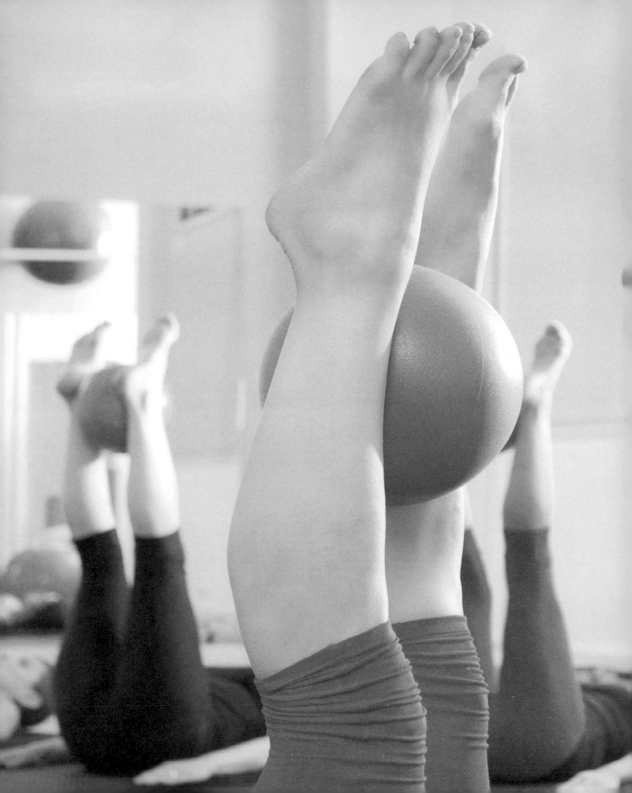

Exercises With Props

Large Pilates Equipment

We have introduced props into your workout to help add interest and variation to your exercises. These are all available through sports stores or online, and all are relatively low priced. However, there are larger, studio-based apparatus which you may come across if you go to special classes.

Common Studio Equipment

Some of the commonest apparatus you may come across are the reformer, the cadillac and the chair. Many instructors also use the barrel to help challenge your range of movement. So what do these pieces of equipment do?

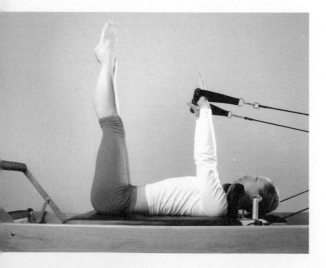

The Reformer

This is the most popular piece of Pilates equipment and one you've probably seen before. This was created by Joseph Pilates and remains unchanged today. It is used in or in similar ways to:

- ✔ **The Hundred (pages 118–19)**
- ✔ **Roll Over (pages 128–30)**
- ✔ **Corkscrew (pages 166–67)**
- ✔ **Jackknife (pages 176–77 and 223)**
- ✔ **Dart (page 97)**
- ✔ **Curl Up (page 91)**
- ✔ **Side Twist (pages 184–85)**
- ✔ **Saw (pages 138–39)**

The Cadillac

This may also be introduced to you as the trapeze table. It looks similar to the pull-down systems you see at many gyms.

This can help you if your spine isn't particularly flexible or you need help stabilizing this area. It is used in or in similar ways to:

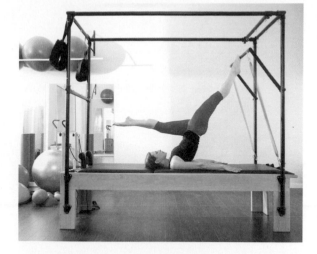

- ✅ **Roll Up (pages 124–25)**
- ✅ **Roll Over (pages 128–30)**
- ✅ **Cat Stretch (page 57)**
- ✅ **Single Leg Stretch (pages 103–04)**
- ✅ **Curl Up (pages 91)**

The Chair

As it says, the chair helps to support you while you perform certain movements, particularly those which may challenge your balance. It is used in or in similar ways to:

- ✅ **Inner Thigh Lift (page 215)**
- ✅ **Torpedo (pages 158–59)**
- ✅ **Roll Down (pages 78–79)**

The Barrel

This piece of equipment provides support for the spine and helps you to improve your core strength. It is used in or in similar ways to:

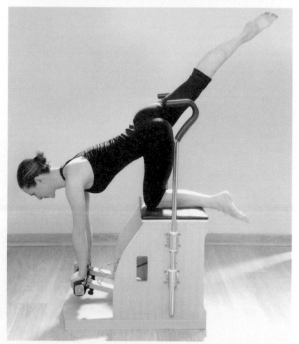

- ✅ **Side Twist (page 184)**
- ✅ **Swan Dive (pages 168–69)**

The Small Ball

Using the ball gives your joints a wonderful massage and support. Take half the air out of the ball to make these movements easier.

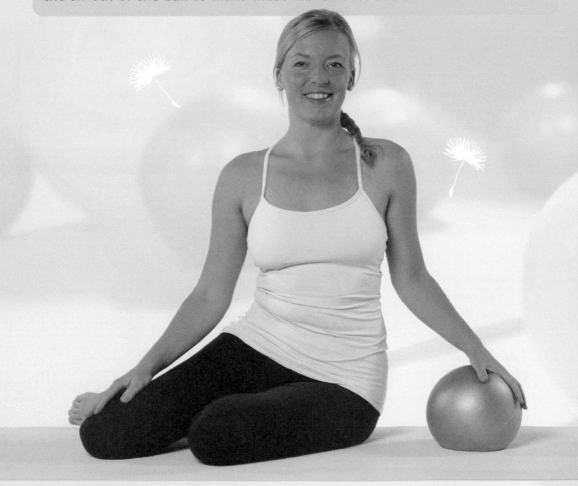

Neck Circles

This movement will help to release any tension around your head and neck area, to improve posture and release any potential headaches.

1 **Lie on the mat** in the starting position. Place your head on the small ball, so that the bottom of the ball sits at the base of your head.

2 **Breathing naturally**, roll your head on the ball in small circular motions, first clockwise and then anti-clockwise.

3 **Begin with large circular movements**, reducing the movements as you go, side to side as though you're saying 'no', then as though you're nodding agreement, then squash the ball into the floor. Go as slowly and controlled as you can.

4 **Repeat** up to **10** times in each direction.

Top Tip

Close your eyes and feel the muscles in your neck, shoulders and spine release.

3

Side Ball Twist

Imagine you're wringing all the water out of the ball as you give your side a wonderful massage and stretch.

1 **Lie on your left side** with the ball under the curve of your waist. Your knees should be on top of each other, feet flexed facing towards the back of the mat.

2 **Breathe in** and, as you exhale, stretch your right leg outwards, toes pointed.

3 **Place your right arm** behind your head, bending at the elbow. Lean on your left arm, which should be propping up your upper body.

4 **Twist forwards**, so that your face moves down towards the mat and your body 'wrings out' the ball.

5 **Reverse the movement**, so that you're facing behind you.

6 Repeat **three** to **five** times.

7 **Repeat** on the opposite side.

Dead Bug On The Ball

This is similar to your arm work, with the added benefit of support under your lower back.

1

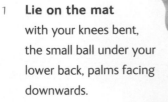

1 **Lie on the mat** with your knees bent, the small ball under your lower back, palms facing downwards.

2 **Breathe in** and, as you exhale, lift your right leg, keeping your toes pointed and knee slightly bent.

2

3 **Still breathing out**, bring
your left leg up to join the right.

4 **Breathe out**, then bring your
right arm up, so that it's parallel
to your knees. Your palm should
be facing inwards.

4

5 **Breathe in** and bring
your other arm up so your
palms are facing, but without
your hands touching.

6 **Hold this position** for the count
of five, then return limb by limb
to the starting position.

5

Side To Side With The Ball

This is a very challenging move that works your entire body. Only complete this move if you feel confident in your strength and stability.

1   **Place the ball** between your feet and lift them to the ceiling. Your arms should be facing down, stretched out to your sides.

2   **Slightly sway your legs** to the right, keeping your focus on your core.

3   **Return to the centre**, then repeat on the opposite side.

4   **Repeat six to eight times** in each direction.

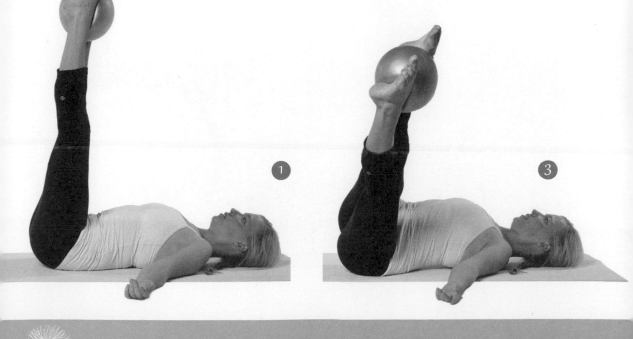

The Magic Circle

The magic circle, or toning circle as it's also known, can help to strengthen and work the inner thighs and arms – notoriously difficult areas to tone.

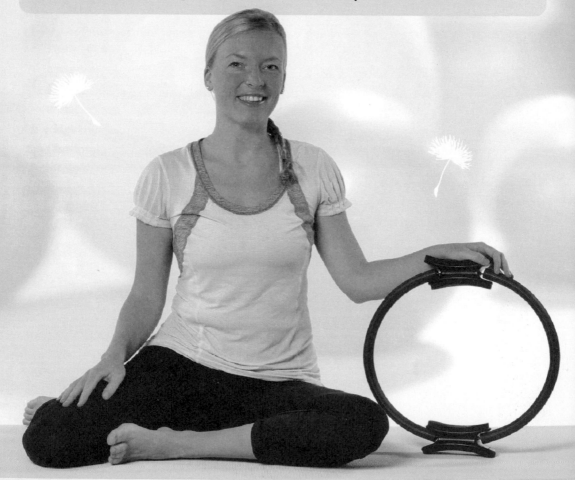

Inner Thigh Squeezes

Work those inner thighs by squeezing the magic circle. Make sure that your hips and spine are stable, so that you don't feel the workout in your lower back.

1   **Start by lying on your back** on the mat with your knees bent and your feet planted on the ground.

2   **Place the magic circle** between your thighs about three inches above the knee.

3   **Inhale to prepare** and then exhale as you squeeze the magic circle with your thighs. Inhale as you release the circle and then exhale as you squeeze again.

4   **Be sure** that these repetitions are slow and controlled.

5   **After 10 squeezes**, hold the magic circle slightly squeezed and then begin a set of 16 pulses.

6   **To finish**, squeeze the magic circle as much as you can and hold it for five breaths.

Top Tip

Try to keep the magic circle slightly squeezed the entire time.

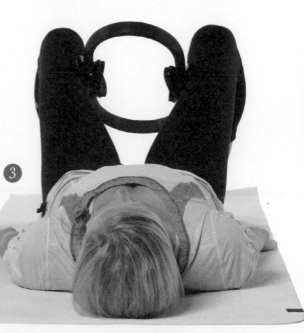

3

Roll Up

Similar to the roll up described on pages 124–25, the added use of the magic circle challenges your core and stability.

1 **Place the magic circle** around one foot and lie back on the mat. Breathe out.

2 **Breathe in** and, activating your core, use your stomach muscles to bring you to a sitting position. You should be able to reach the magic circle now.

3 **Lean forwards**, so that you can feel a stretch in the back of your thigh.

4 **Still holding on to the circle**, slowly return to sitting position, straightening your arms as you go. You probably won't be able to return to the full prone position, so go as far as you can.

5 **Return to the sitting position**, using your stomach muscles, not the circle, to pull you upwards.

6 Repeat **three** to **five** times on the right leg before repeating on the left leg.

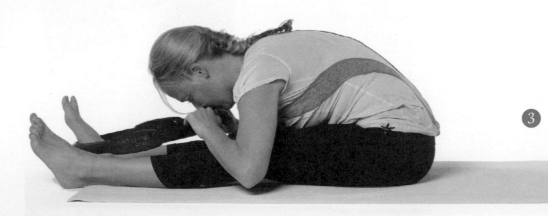

3

Inner Thigh Lift

A wonderful way to stretch your thigh, as well as your lower back and hip joints. Make sure you don't hunch over – keep your posture strong.

1   **Lie on your back** with the magic circle in one hand.

2   **Breathe in and then breathe out**, lifting your right leg to the ceiling, so that as you lift your torso you can place the magic circle around your foot. Make sure that the padded area is around the base of your foot for comfort.

3   **Breathe in and, as you exhale**, return your torso to the mat; your leg should follow your progress, towards your head, as you gently use the magic circle to help yourself downwards.

4   **Repeat five times** on the right leg before swapping over and repeating on the left leg.

Torpedo

A great way to tone those inner thighs as well as reinforcing the stretch and stability in your spinal area.

1   **Lie on your left side** on the mat, with your head resting on your outstretched left arm. The magic circle should be placed between your legs, around your lower calves.

2   **Breathe in to prepare**, feeling your legs take control of the magic circle.

3   **Breathe out** and, from your abominals, lift your legs towards the ceiling, squeezing the magic circle between your legs as you do so. This is a difficult move, so only lift as far as you can. You may also find that you experience cramp in your leg, so just take it slowly.

4   **Hold this lifted position** for two to three breaths before slowly returning to the starting position.

5   **Repeat five times** before repeating the movement on the other side.

Top Tip

Make sure that you don't slump forwards, so use your top arm to support your body and posture.

Roll Over

This is a great all-over workout – it helps to strengthen your entire body, while challenging the stability of your hips and spine.

1   **Lie in the starting position.**
    Take a couple of breaths to prepare.

2   **Stretch forwards** to place the magic circle between your legs, bending your knees up to make it easier. Ensure that the padded sections are comfortably positioned.

3   **Lower your legs**, so that you're back in the starting position, but with the magic circle just above your ankles.

4   **Breathe in** and bring your legs towards the ceiling, keeping your torso still and activated.

Top Tip

Make sure that you're not using your arms or your hands to lift your legs up. They should be loosely placed on the mat, not pressing hard into the floor. Use your abdominal muscles for this movement.

3

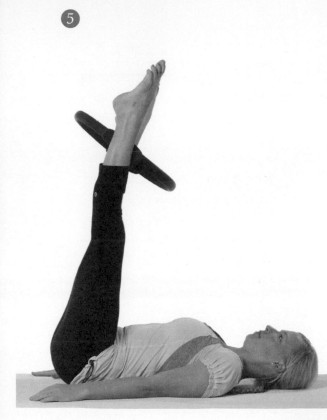

5 **Breathe out** as your legs continue to lift up and over your head, while keeping the magic circle firmly between your legs.

6 **As you continue** to lift your legs, your pelvis and spine will automatically follow. Keep your movements steady.

7 **Breathe in** and continue to lower your legs behind you until, ideally, your toes are almost touching the mat.

8 **Breathe out** and, using your core strength, lift your legs back to the starting position, taking it as slowly as possible.

9 **Repeat** up to **five** times.

Stretch Band

These stretchy, rubbery bands can be used in most exercise classes, and even yoga classes. However, with the introduction of props such as the magic circle, stretch bands do not tend to be used as often as they once were.

A stretch band provides extra resistance to your Pilates workout, and can help to tone your arms, legs, core muscles, lower back, hips and abdominals. If you're doing the workout at home and you don't have a magic circle, you can use a stretch band in most of the magic circle exercises instead, to create a similar workout environment.

Exercises you can incorporate a stretch band into include the following – ask your Pilates instructor:

- **Standing Leg Press**
- **Oblique Twist**
- **Waist Twist (similar to Spine Twist, page 136)**
- **Roll Downs (page 78–79)**

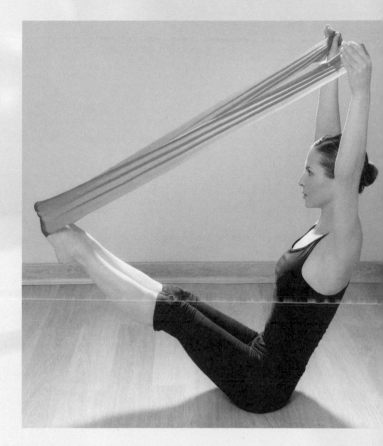

The Pilates Ball

The Pilates Ball, also known as an exercise ball or Swiss ball, helps to promote stability and utilize your stomach muscles. It's great for pregnant women, as it takes the pressure away from the lower back.

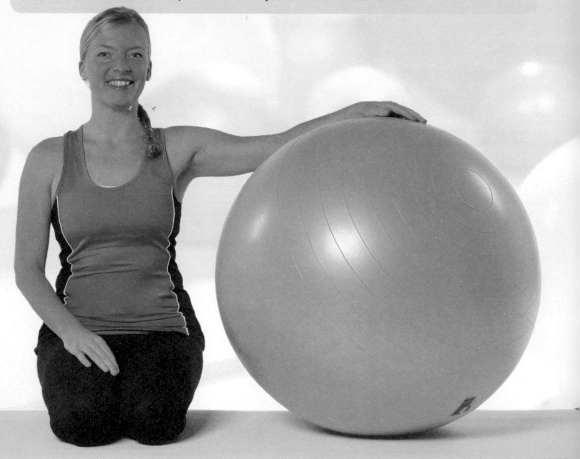

Side To Side

Open up the hips and relax the lower back with this great stretch, which helps reinforce your stability.

1 **Lie on your back** with your arms at your sides, palms facing upwards. Place a Pilates ball under your thighs, so that your knees are bent.

2 **Breathe in** and enforce the feeling of hugging the ball with your legs, while maintaining a strong and firm core.

3 **Breathe out** and slowly roll your legs to the side. Your right hip will lift slightly, although your torso and head should remain still.

4 **Breathe in** and return your legs to the middle, before rolling towards the right side.

5 **Repeat** the movement **five** to **eight** times.

Hamstring Curl

This is a great move to open up the lower back and increase the flexibility in your knees. If you regularly run or sit at a desk for long hours, this will help to stretch your legs.

1　**Lie on the mat** with your lower legs placed on the exercise ball. Your arms should be stretched out to your sides. Breathe in to prepare.

2　**Raise your back and hips** off the floor, while straightening your lower back, knees and hips out in front of you. The ball should move slightly forwards and you'll need to press down slightly on the ball with your feet to control it. Keep your spine and pelvis strong and stable. Hold here for three seconds, breathing normally.

3　**Breathe in**, then, as you exhale, bring the ball back towards your body. Your feet will lower on the ball, so that your feet are flat. Your spine and bottom will lower slightly towards the ground, but not all the way. Hold here and take a couple of breaths.

4　Repeat **five** times.

3

Jackknife

This move is a lot of fun, although be warned: you will probably fall off the ball until you master the exercise. It's a great way to massage your torso and open up the muscles in your back.

1   **Kneel on the mat** with the ball in front of you. Steady it with your right hand.

2   **Lift yourself up and on to the ball**, resting on your stomach, bending your elbows to balance. Your feet should be flexed. Take a breath in to prepare and to stabilize your position on the ball.

3   **Breathe out** and push yourself off from your feet, so that your body rides up and over the ball. Reach forwards with your hands to rest your upper body on your outstretched arms. One hand will be slightly in front of the other.

4   **Hold the position** here and breathe deeply. Using your abdominal muscles, pull your knees in under your chest, before pushing back until your legs are fully extended. Repeat **five** to **ten** times.

5   **Return to step 2**, using your hands to push you back.

3

Pike

One of the most difficult moves, it can take some practice to do this movement without falling off! Keep at it though, and you'll feel a great sense of achievement.

1 **Begin on all fours**, with your knees bent on the ball, your outstretched arms supporting your upper body. Make sure you don't lock out your elbows. Your feet should be pointed. Breathe in to prepare yourself.

2 **Exhale and, using your legs**, not your lower back, pull your legs forwards, so that you're in a crouched position in front of the ball, your hips almost directly over your shoulders. Your arms are still straight, but your upper body has lowered slightly towards the floor.

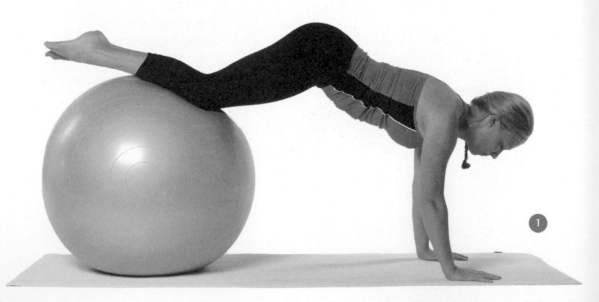

1

3   **Inhale as you push** the ball to the back of the mat. Your back should be straight and your legs and toes pointed.

4   **Exhale and bring the ball forwards again** until your torso is vertical, your shoulders and hips in alignment. Your upper body should be in a handstand position, with your legs lowered on to the ball, resting on your pointed toes.

5   **Check that your torso is stable**, your abdominals are strong, and your hips and pelvis are stable.

6   **Inhale and slowly lower yourself** back towards the floor, so that the ball rolls backwards until you're in step 3 position.

7   Repeat **three** to **five** times.

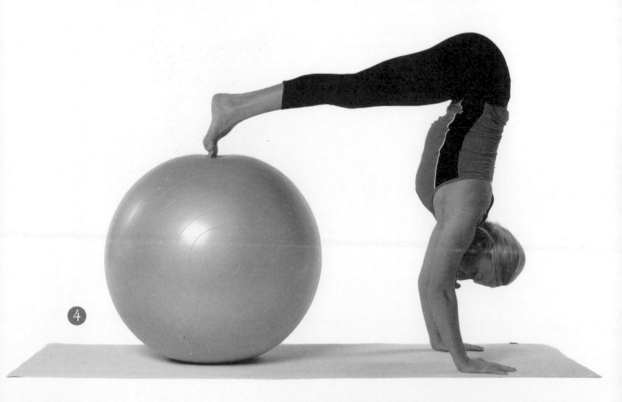

The Foam Roller

These are wonderful pieces of equipment to help detoxify your body and give you a specific body massage. Be warned, they may look soft, but the massage can be quite painful as it works away at any knots and tight spots.

Illiotibial Band (ITB) Massage

This is a wonderful massage for the outsides of your thighs. It helps to remove toxins and massage any sore muscles in your thighs.

1 **Place the foam roller** under your ITB (outer thigh). Using your arms, very slowly move your body over the roller and back, allowing it to massage the outer thigh.

2 **Breathe normally** and keep your legs relaxed.

3 This can feel **slightly painful** to start with, but it will ease off.

4 **Repeat** this process for 15–90 seconds.

5 **Swap legs** and repeat on the other leg.

Top Tip

This exercise can be performed with both legs off the ground as per the image, or with the upper leg in contact with the ground (via the foot) in front of or behind the lower leg, whichever is more comfortable.

Gluteal Massage

This may feel slightly painful, but try to remember that it's a good pain as the roller massages your thighs and glutes.

1 **Sit on your roller** with your knees bent, leaning on your arms. Your hands and fingers should be pointing to the back of the mat.

2 **Lift your left leg** and rest your ankle on your right knee, so that your left leg forms a triangle shape.

3 **Use the stability** of the bent right leg to push yourself backwards on the roller until the roller is under your bottom. Return to the start and repeat **five** to **seven** times. Repeat on the opposite leg.

Top Tip

If this doesn't feel like it's giving your glutes a sufficiently deep massage, you can replace the foam roller with a tennis ball. But be warned! It'll hurt!

Upper Back Massage

Release the tensions of the day and from your workout with this wonderfully relaxing upper-back massage. This is also a good movement to do at the end of the day, even if it's the only Pilates exercise you have time for.

1   **Sit on your mat** with your knees slightly bent and the foam roller placed under your shoulder blades. Your hands should be behind your head, as though you're doing a sit-up.

2   **Slowly lower your upper body** down on to the roller, so that you achieve a lovely curve in your spine.

3   **Using your abdominal muscles,** lift your torso and bottom off the floor.

This will automatically push the roller further back under your shoulders. Hold this position and feel your muscles relax on to the roller.

Top Tip

Take this as slowly as possible. Don't worry if you hear cracking or crunching noises, it's just your spine getting into the correct position!

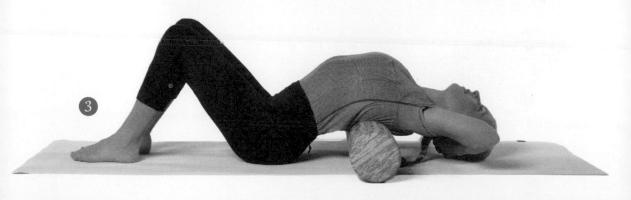

Massaging Upper Back And Shoulders

This is a continuation of the previous movement, focusing on relaxing the neck, upper back and shoulder muscles.

1 **Repeat the steps** in Upper Back Massage on page 229.

2 **Continue the relaxing movement** by pushing further down on your feet, so that the roller now reaches under your neck and shoulders.

3 **Relax here for a while**, allowing your neck and shoulders to sink into the foam. Lightly roll the roller back and forth under your neck and shoulders to give yourself a mini massage.

Arm Reaches

Massage your spine and open your chest area with this stretch, which helps to remind you to stabilize your spine and pelvis area.

1   **Place your foam roller** so that it's lengthways on your mat.

2   **Lie on the roller**, feet flat on the floor, so that the length of the roller mirrors your spine. Your head should also be resting on the roller.

3   **Lift your arms** above you, keeping your shoulder blades down. Your palms should be facing each other.

4   **Lower your arms** to either side of your body. You'll need to maintain a stable spine and pelvis for this movement so that you don't fall off the roller.

5   **Sweep your arms** backwards until they're behind your head, fingertips (possibly) touching the ground.

6   **Return to** the starting position. Repeat **three** to **five** times.

Top Tip

You can increase your stability by raising your knees 90 degrees to the mat. Balancing on the roller will test the strength of your core.

4

Dead Bug Balance

The description says it all. Balancing on the foam roller will take some time, stability and strength. It's a great way to challenge your pelvic stability, while giving the muscles on either side of your spine a massage.

1 **Lie on the foam roller** with your knees bent and in the air at slightly more than a 90-degree angle, arms by your sides.

2 **Breathe in and focus** on balancing on the mat, using your abdominal muscles to push your body on to the roller.

3 **Breathe out** and lift your left arm up, so that your arm is in front of your shoulder

4 **Continue to exhale** and bring your right arm up so that your palms are facing each other

5 **Remain here** for a couple of breaths before returning your right arm to the floor, followed by the left arm.

6 Repeat **three** to **five** times, then swap the order of the arms.

3

Checklist

Large Pilates Equipment

- [ ] The Reformer
- [ ] The Cadillac
- [ ] The Chair
- [ ] The Barrel

The Small Ball

- [ ] Neck Circles
- [ ] Side Ball Twist
- [ ] Dead Bug On The Ball
- [ ] Side To Side With The Ball

The Magic Circle

- [ ] Inner Thigh Squeezes
- [ ] Roll Up
- [ ] Inner Thigh Lift
- [ ] Preparation For Camel
- [ ] Roll Over

The Stretch Band

- [ ] Standing Leg Press
- [ ] Oblique Twist
- [ ] Waist Twist
- [ ] Roll Downs

The Pilates Ball

- [ ] Side To Side
- [ ] Hamstring Curl
- [ ] Jackknife
- [ ] Pike

The Foam Roller

- [ ] Illiotibial Band (ITB) Massage
- [ ] Gluteal Massage
- [ ] Upper Back Massage
- [ ] Massaging Upper Back And Shoulders
- [ ] Arm Reaches
- [ ] Dead Bug Balance

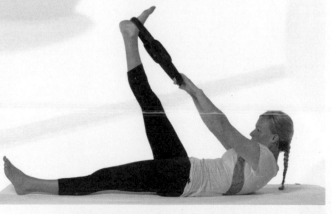

Routines
For You

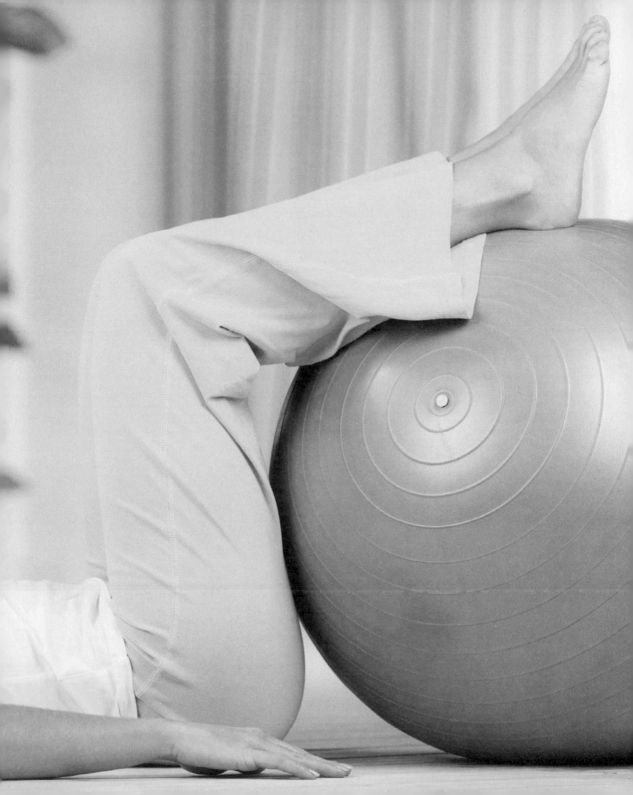

Pilates Sequences

Find a routine that suits your physical needs and requirements, whether it's a bad back, lack of energy or perhaps a lack of time.

All-Rounder Moves

Ideally, incorporate Introduction To Your Stability (pages 54–65), Basic Standing Exercises (pages 66–79) and Basic Mat Exercises (pages 80–115) into your everyday routine. These give you a good grounding and knowledge of the foundations of Pilates and will help you to practise your core stability. As you become more confident with the moves, you may pick and choose from the other movements, especially from the more difficult sections.

The following Pilates routines have been designed with one thing in mind: your optimal health. While we are all busy and have very little time to exercise, you can do just 15 minutes of Pilates exercises a day (Daily Maintenance, pages 238–50) and still achieve some health and fitness benefits.

For Specific Health Concerns

We have selected the routines with the commonest health issues in mind: stress, weight problems, back pain and tiredness. According to the World Health Organization (WHO), taking just 30 minutes of your day and dedicating it to exercise can help to prevent many health issues facing the Western world.

You don't have to choose just the one routine! Incorporate one, two or all of the routines together, depending on your time, experience and energy levels. Whatever you choose, enjoy!

There is no set order in which you must complete the exercises listed in any routine, though they do follow a natural progression in terms of difficulty.

Daily Maintenance

These movements should be done, as the name suggests, every day, to help confirm your core strength and to help your body get into the habit of stretching and moving every day.

- ✅ **Cat Stretch** (page 57)
- ✅ **Setting Up** (page 56)
- ✅ **Single Knee Opening** (page 60)
- ✅ **Imprinting** (page 63)
- ✅ **Toe Taps** (page 239)
- ✅ **Curl Ups** (page 91)
- ✅ **Oblique Curl Ups** (page 92)
- ✅ **Hip Rolls** (page 93)
- ✅ **Shoulder Bridge** (page 174)
- ✅ **Bridge** (page 87)
- ✅ **Back Extension** (page 140)
- ✅ **Diamond Press** (page 96)
- ✅ **Superman** (page 240)
- ✅ **Book Opening (Lying)** (page 100)
- ✅ **Side Leg Lift** (page 241)

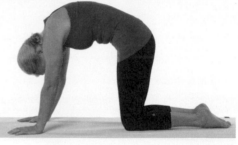

Cat Stretch

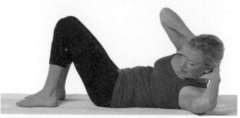

Oblique Curl Ups

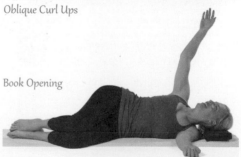

Book Opening

Toe Taps

Practise your stability and strengthen your core with this relaxing movement.

1   **Lie down on your mat** with your knees bent, arms to your sides.

2   **Breathe in**, activating your pelvic floor.

3   **Slowly lift your left leg**, keeping the knee bent, until it's 90 degrees to your mat with your shin parallel to the floor. Keep it there for the count of three.

4   **Now lift your right leg** to join your left leg. Maintain this pose for another few breaths.

5   **Lower your left leg** so that your toe is 'tapping' the mat, keeping stable through your pelvis and spine. Bring it back up and do the same with the right leg. Continue, taking turns with each leg.

Top Tip

If this movement hurts your lower back, don't lift your leg up so high. Place a pillow under your head to relieve any further pressure.

5

Superman

Increase your co-ordination and core control with this super move.

1 **Begin on all fours**, with your hands under your shoulders and knees under your hips.

2 **Draw in your pelvic floor** and lower tummy.

3 **Slowly extend the opposite arm** and leg away from the body. Keep everything still except the limbs that are extending away.

4 **Ensure that your chin** is tucked in and you feel the stretch through the length of your spine.

5 **Alternate sides** until you've done **ten** movements on each side.

Top Tip

If you're wobbling out of control, first lift your leg, and stabilize your position before lifting the opposite arm.

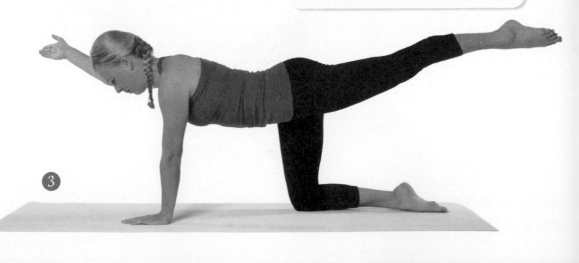

Side Leg Lift

Strengthen your gluteal muscles and stabilize your hips. This will help to avoid and prevent any lower back pain.

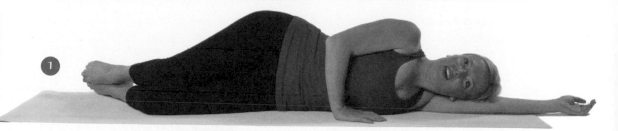

1. **Lie on your side** with your legs bent and your left arm stretched straight out to the end of the mat.

2. **Draw in** your pelvic floor and core.

3. **Lengthen the top leg** away from the body, then lift it to hip height only. Gently lower the leg.

4. **Repeat 20 times**, then repeat on the opposite side.

Top Tip

Make sure that your pelvis doesn't move backwards, as this is cheating and you won't receive the full benefits of the move.

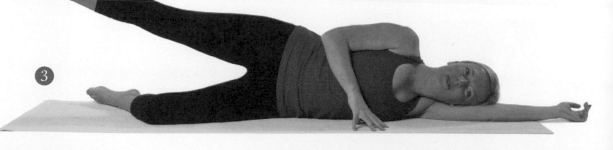

To Strengthen Abdominals

Achieve hard abdominals as well as minimize your stomach fat with the following exercises. They'll help to stabilize your hips and spine as well as remind you to activate your core and keep a strong centre throughout the day.

- **Pelvic Clocks** (page 84)
- **Pelvic Rolls** (page 86)
- **Hip Rolls** (page 93)
- **Curl Ups** (page 91)
- **The Hundred** (page 118)
- **Single Leg Stretch** (page 103)
- **Double Leg Stretch** (page 109)
- **Mermaid** (page 162)
- **Dart** (page 97)
- **Torpedo** (page 158)
- **Rolling Like A Ball** (page 133)
- **Scissors** (page 120)

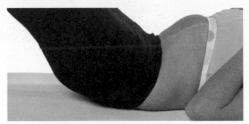

Pelvic Rolls

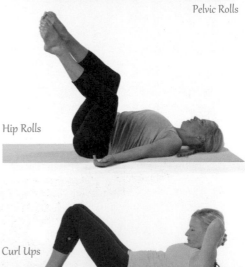

Hip Rolls

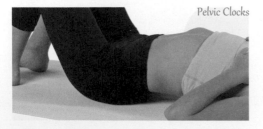

Pelvic Clocks

Curl Ups

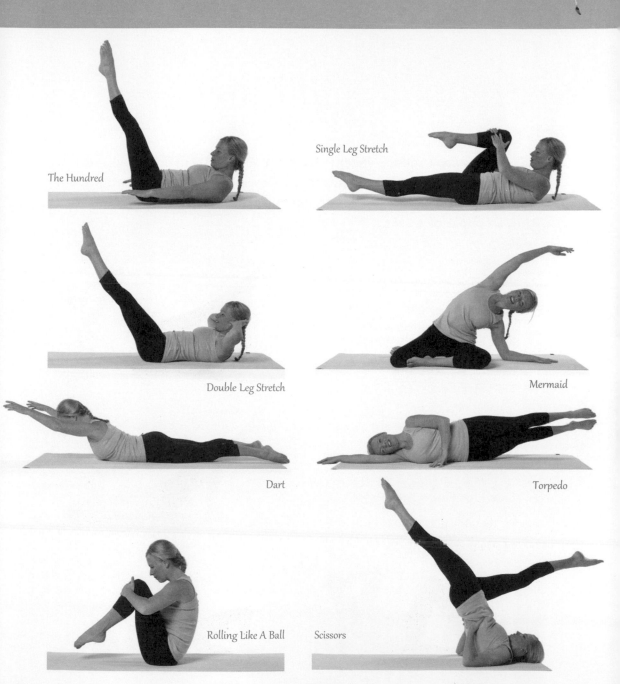

The Hundred

Single Leg Stretch

Double Leg Stretch

Mermaid

Dart

Torpedo

Rolling Like A Ball

Scissors

For Bums And Thighs

While Pilates can't reduce specific fat from your bottom and thighs, it can help to tone and lift this area with the following exercises. Be patient, but you should begin to notice a difference in this area, with daily workouts, within a couple of weeks.

- **Pelvic Clocks** (page 84)
- **Side Plank Leg Lift** (page 148)
- **Side Kick Series: Up and Down** (page 152)
- **Side Kick Series: Front and Back** (page 150)
- **Clam** (page 111)
- **Bridge** (page 87)
- **Side Kick Series: Side Passé** (page 178)
- **Leg Pull Front** (page 245)

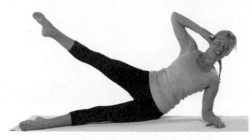

Side Kick Series: Up and Down

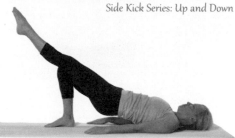

Bridge

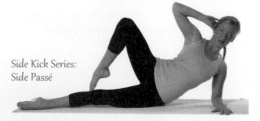

Side Kick Series: Side Passé

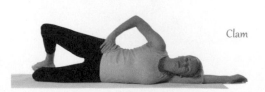

Clam

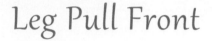

Leg Pull Front

Stretch your legs and create a long, lean look with this move.

1 **Sit with your legs extended**, your hands on the floor either side of your body, fingers pointing inwards.

2 **Lift your hips** off the floor, bringing your body into a straight line.

3 **Raise your left leg** as high as you can, toes pointed, without moving your hips. Keep these firm and stable.

4 **Hold** for the count of three.

5 **Return to the starting position** and repeat on the opposite side.

6 **Continue to repeat** on each side, up to **five** times on each.

For Toned Arms

If you're struck with the dreaded bingo wings, you'll know how difficult it is to tone the lower muscles in your arms. As we age, the skin and muscles in this area become looser, but the following moves will reignite the strength in this area.

- ☑ **Arm Circles** (page 83)
- ☑ **Table Top** (page 94)
- ☑ **Stingray** (page 156)
- ☑ **Swimming** (page 160)
- ☑ **Plank Leg Pull Back** (page 247)
- ☑ **Side Twist** (page 184)
- ☑ **Side Plank** (page 147)

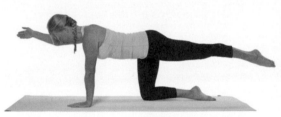

Table Top

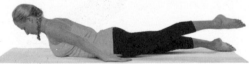

Stingray

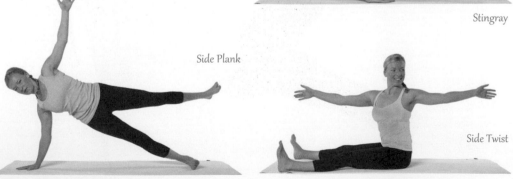

Side Plank

Side Twist

Plank Leg Pull Back

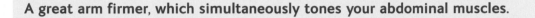

A great arm firmer, which simultaneously tones your abdominal muscles.

1   **Get into plank position** with your hands placed evenly under your shoulders and your toes pointed. Your back should be straight, not curved or lifted.

2   **Breathe in** and strengthen and stabilize your core.

3   **Breathe out** and slowly lift your left leg towards the ceiling. Your toes should be pointed downwards, so that your foot is flexed. Keep your head stable, so that you're looking straight down at your mat.

4   **Hold this position** for a count, then return to the start. Repeat **five** times on the left leg before repeating the movement on the right leg.

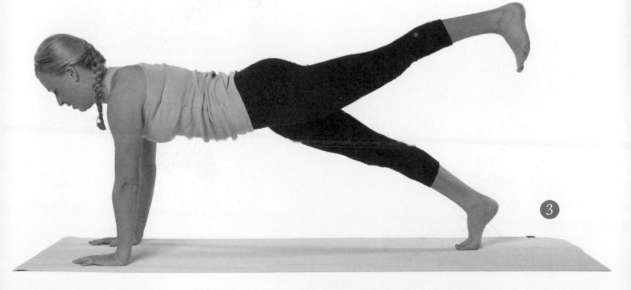

Pilates For Energy

Whether you need to rev your energy levels up a gear for the day ahead, or you need an afternoon boost, these exercises will leave you feeling recharged and revitalized.

- ☑ **Tennis Ball Rising** (page 70)
- ☑ **Roll Down** (page 78)
- ☑ **Bridge** (page 87)
- ☑ **The Hundred** (page 118)
- ☑ **Open Leg Rocker** (page 135)
- ☑ **Spine Stretch** (page 126)
- ☑ **Saw** (page 138)
- ☑ **Scissors** (page 120)
- ☑ **Bicycle** (page 172)

Bridge

Saw

Bicycle

Troubleshooting

Pilates, like all exercises, should be avoided at certain times. If you are afflicted by particular injuries or if you have a pre-existing medical condition, you may not be able to do all the recommended exercises. Alternatively, you may be able to perform modified versions of them.

Pregnancy

Pilates is an ideal form of exercise both during and after pregnancy. However, it's recommended that you don't participate in Pilates classes during your first trimester, particularly if you haven't done classes before. It's best to check with your GP, obstetrician and Pilates instructor before you begin. When you do attend classes, you should be aware of the following issues:

✔ **Some of the positions**, especially those lying on your tummy or back, or standing on one leg, are not suitable for mid-pregnancy and beyond. Your instructor will advise you on which ones are recommended for you and will give you alternatives to try instead.

✔ **Avoid stretching any joints to their full range**. This is because the hormone relaxin that is released during pregnancy will make your ligaments looser. So you may feel more flexible, but, in this case, going to your edge might lead to overextension and injury.

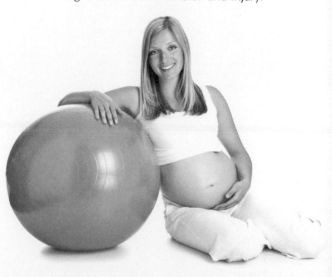

❖ **Many pregnant and post-natal women** suffer from carpal tunnel syndrome, which can be immensely painful in the knees and wrists. Positions that require you to support your weight on your knees and hands are not advised. Instead, you may need to lean forwards on a Swiss ball.

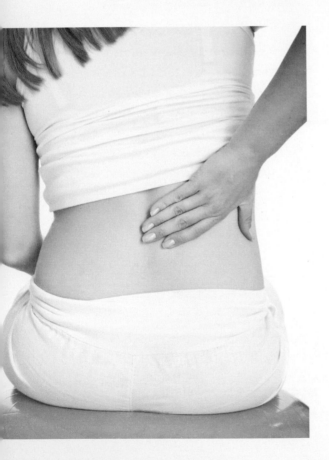

Back Pain

While Pilates is ideal for those suffering from back pain, there are some instances where a class is not ideal, or where you would derive greater benefit from one-on-one supervision. If you've been in an accident, had surgery on your back, suffered a slipped disc or nerve damage, it's best to speak to your GP and instructor before you begin. A properly trained Pilates teacher will be able to advise you on the best exercise routine for you, and adapt movements as necessary.

Weight Loss

Although Pilates can help to encourage you to lead a healthier lifestyle, it's not a cardiovascular workout. This means that your heart rate won't dramatically increase, so you won't be burning up large amounts of energy. In order to lose weight, you need to burn more calories than you eat. If you're serious about weight loss, the best approach is to speak to your GP. Pilates can certainly be part of a healthier regime, along with regular walking, swimming, cycling or aerobics classes.

Checklist

☐ **Daily maintenance:** Using exercises such as Cat Stretch and Hip Rolls, improve your core strength and get your body used to stretching and moving every day. Just 15–30 minutes of these movements will help you to incorporate a great Pilates habit into your life.

☐ **To strengthen abdominals:** For many women, their abdominals can become weakened as they age or after childbirth. Movements such as the Hundred and Rolling Like a Ball are great ab strengtheners.

☐ **For bums and thighs:** The most hated area by many women (whether it's justified or not!), these movements, such as Side Kicks and Clams, are hard to do, but well worth the effort, as they tone and strengthen these areas.

☐ **For toned arms:** As we age, the muscles in our upper arms become weakened, leaving us with 'tuckshop lady' arms (or 'bingo wings'). Prevent this sagging by incorporating movements such as Arm Circles and Side Plank into your routine. They look easy, but the benefits are long-reaching.

☐ **Pilates for energy:** Whether it's the start of the day, or you need a quick pick-me-up, these exercises, including Tennis Ball Rising and Spine Stretch, help to increase the blood flow throughout your body and help you to clear and focus your mind.

☐ **Troubleshooting:** Pilates is an ideal form of exercise to help prevent illness and injury. However, if you're pregnant, have injuries or medical problems such as osteoporosis, it's important that you speak to your instructor or GP before doing certain exercises. And remember, if you feel any twinge of pain, stop, breathe and take a break.

Further Reading

Bussell, D., *Pilates for Life*, Michael Joseph, 2005

Campbell, M., *Pilates on the Go*, Hodder & Stoughton, 2012

Cathie, K. and Robinson, L., *The Pilates Bible. The Most Comprehensive and Accessible Guide to Pilates Ever*, Kyle Cathie, 2010

Craig, C., *Pilates on the Ball: The World's Most Popular Workout Using the Exercise Ball*, Healing Arts Press. Inner Traditions, 2001

Ferris, J., *The Pilates Bible: The Definitive Guide to Pilates Exercises*, Goldsfield Press, 2013

Gillies, L., *101 Ways to Work Out on the Ball: Sculpt Your Ideal Body with Pilates, Yoga and More*, Fair Winds Press, 2004

Herman, E., *Pilates for Dummies*, John Wiley & Sons, 2002

Herman, E., *Pilates Matwork Props Workbook. Illustrated Step-by-step Guide*, Ulysses Press, 2004

Isacowitz, R., *Pilates*, Human Kinetics Europe Ltd., 2006

Kent, A., *PILATES: Annabel Kent's Six Minute Life-Changing Routine*, The Electronic Book Company. 2013 (Kindle Only)

Lawrence, D., *Pilates Method: An Integrative Approach to Teaching (Fitness Professionals)*. A&C Black Publishers Ltd, 2008

Lyon, D., *The Complete Book of Pilates for Men*. Regan Books, 2005

Massey, P., *Sports Pilates*, CICO Books, 2011

Paterson, J., *Teaching Pilates for Postural Faults. Illness and Injury: A Practical Guide*, Butterworth-Heinemann, 2008

Pilates, J. and Miller, W., *A Pilates' Primer: Return to Life through Contrology and Your Health*, Presentation Dynamics Inc, 2000

Pilates, J. and Miller, W., *A Pilates Primer: Return to Life through Contrology and Your Health, Revised Edition for the 21st Century*, Presentation Dynamics Inc, 2012

Robinson, L., Fisher, H., Knox, J. and Thomson, G., *The Official Body Control Pilates Manual: The Ultimate Guide to the Pilates Method – For Fitness, Health. Sport and at Work*, Pan, 2002

Robinson, L., Fisher, H. and Massey, P., *The Body Control Pilates Back Book*, Pan, 2002

Selby, A., *Pilates for a Flat Stomach: Perfect Abs in Just 15 Minutes a Day*, Thorsons, 2003

Ungaro, A., *Pilates: Body in Motion*, Dorling Kindersley, 2002

Ungaro, A., *15 Minute Everyday Pilates: Get Real Results Anytime, Anywhere, Four 15-minute Workouts*. Dorling Kindersley, 2008

Websites

www.australianpilates.asn.au
A not-for-profit Australian Pilates representative body. this website allows you to find a Pilates instructor in Australia as well as offering comprehensive information on how to become a Pilates teacher yourself.

www.bodycontrolpilates.com
Body Control Pilates is an established website, useful if you are looking for a Pilates teacher or are interested in training as one.

www.corepilates.co.nz
Providing information on Stott Pilates, Core Pilates Studio, New Zealand, offers personalized Pilates sessions to help with injury rehabilitation and general wellbeing.

www.homehealthpilates.co.uk
This website offers convenient home and park Pilates services on either a one-to-one or small group basis in London, UK with experienced instructors.

www.merrithew.com
A great website that helps you find highly trained Pilates instructors in the US as well as a useful online shop for all your equipment needs.

www.nhs.uk/Livewell/fitness/Pages/pilates.aspx
An informative site if you're unsure if Pilates is for you, you can take a look at what the medical community has to say about Pilates.

www.pilates.co.uk
The ultimate Pilates reference site, with links to the wider global Pilates community.

www.pilatesalliance.net
An interesting website that provides information on the practices of Pilates Alliance Australia who act as a regulatory body for control of quality instruction and member support within all legitimate approaches to the Pilates Method.

www.pilatesfoundation.com
A non-profit organization that supports the teaching of Pilates across the UK.

www.pilates-mad.com
A great site for those mad about having the correct Pilates equipment, a comprehensive range of mats. gym balls and other Pilates equipment.

www.pilatesmethodalliance.org
This website offers information around The Pilates Method Alliance which is the professional association and certifying agency for Pilates in the US.

www.pilatesnearyou.co.uk
A great site if you are looking for a Pilates instructor. studio or class in the UK.

www.pilatesunion.com
A great UK-based website, Pilates Union® offers information on all things Pilates related, such as teacher training, instructor directories and equipment sales.

www.polestarpilates.co.nz
Polestar Education is a worldwide provider of rehabilitation-based Pilates curriculum, high-calibre Pilates teachers and successful Pilates studio prototypes.

www.thelivingwellstudio.com.au
An interesting website that offers a holistic approach to the wellbeing of individuals through the practice of Pilates, massage and physiotherapy.

www.themethodpilates.ca
A comprehensive website that offers a range of Pilates teacher training programmes and instruction in Pilates across Canada.

www.unitedstatespilatesassociation.com
The United States Pilates Association offers a comprehensive guide to all aspects of Pilates teacher training.

Index